Design Control, Medical Device Risk and Medical Device Regulation (MDR 2017/745)

An Integrated Approach for Medical Devices

Des O'Brien © 2020

ISBN: 9798690205256
Imprint: Independently published

Contents

APPENDIX 1

Regulation (EU) 2017/745—Listed Summary of Chapters and Articles

Foreword

This short book is a starting point to introduce design control, risk management, regulatory impact and application of Medical Device Directive MDR 2017/745, or to give its full name Regulation (EU) 2017/745 of The European Parliament and of The Council of 5 April 2017 on Medical Devices, Amending Directive 2001/83/EC, Regulation (EC) No. 178/2002 and Regulation (EC) No 1223/2009 and Repealing Council Directives 90/385/EEC and 93/42/EEC.

The importance of design controls manifests itself in the potential impact of device quality and safety for the public or patient in need of medical devices or therapeutic devices. The benefits of well-executed design controls support a device and product development life cycle that ensures the intended use is met and verified during the product development process and beyond. Best practice and compliant application of design controls depend on input definition, appropriate review of inputs and continuous verification and validation to provide outputs. Design control regulations ensure that good quality management (QM) practices are used for the design of medical devices and products remain fit for purpose and appropriate to the intended use.

Adding to the design control requirements for manufacturers is the science of risk management applied to devices and products across the life cycle of each product.

Risk needs to be a continuous consideration and is not just a static or once-off activity. The approach to risk must be suitable for the device in question. A risk plan should lay out the approach, requirements and techniques used to assess risk and complete risk analysis. Any risks that remain must have a clinical benefit and must be managed to ensure residual risks are as low as possible. Therefore, an integrated approach to design, risk management and manufacturing creates a template for safe and effective products.

Recent regulatory requirements that will shape the future of medical device regulation have gained increasing importance. One such regulation is the medical device regulation prescribed by the European Union, MDR 2017/745 and associated amendments. These requirements shape the manner of an organisation's management of risk and the safety of users. Any risk assessments depend on the design features of a device, and how well they are implemented, verified and validated. Only a well-planned and well-maintained quality management system, cognizant of regulation, design management and risk management will achieve compliance and success.

Part I: Design Control

Part I: Design Control

Introduction

Design controls for medical devices are subject to change management regulations and GMP requirements. Therefore, within the quality management system structures, changes must be documented, reviewed and approved to maintain the validated state. In product development, often it takes multiple iterations of designs before a design is selected that meets all of the inputs and stakeholder needs. This iterative process must be documented and controlled to ensure consistent development and ultimately alignment of design inputs and outputs. Design control and change management instil good engineering practice, project management, the cross-functional performance of teams, compliance to legal and regulatory requirements and works to ensure that key critical performance and safety requirements are documented and controlled during the development and indeed throughout the life cycle of the product.

Design controls are prescribed by regulatory authorities and standards such as ISO 13485. However, the focus of teams should go beyond the legal responsibilities and work to ensure safe and reliable products reach patients and users. A measure of this success is the fulfilment of user needs and design inputs via outputs.

Regulatory guidance is largely drawn upon the FDA 21 CFR 820.30, Design Control. In addition to FDA 21 CFR 820.30, a guidance document for medical device manufacturers was issued in 1997. (Reference, Design Control Guidance For Medical Device Manufacturers, March 1997.) ISO 13485 also calls for the product realisation process to include design changes per clause 7. Compliance to ISO 13485 is a fundamental requirement and represents a state of the art application of design and development and product realisation.

Design controls are often described as an interrelated set of practices and procedures that are incorporated into the design and development process, via reviews, cross-functional alignment and a step-by-step roadmap, ensuring that a systematic assessment of the design is an integral part of development. The goal, therefore, is to identify gaps in design inputs and requirements and to highlight any misalignment in the design versus outcome to ensure they are addressed early on in the process.

Key Benefits

- Visibility of requirements versus outputs
- Design focus
- Resource alignment
- Compliance to regulations
- Early recognition of design issues

CFR - Code of Federal Regulations Title 21

FDA requirements provide a structured roadmap to design controls for medical devices:

Design and development (D&D) planning
Design input(s)
Design output(s)
Design review(s)
Design verification
Design validation
Design transfer
Design change management (changes post-transfer managed under change control)
Design History File (DHF)

(a) General states (1) Each manufacturer of any of class III or class II device, and the class I devices listed in paragraph (a)(2) of this section, shall establish and maintain procedures to control the design of the device/product to ensure that specified design requirements are met.

(b) Design and development planning: Each manufacturer shall establish and maintain plans that describe or reference the design and development activities and define responsibility for implementation. The plans shall identify and describe the interfaces with different groups or activities that provide, or result in, input to the design and development process. The plans shall be reviewed, updated, and approved as design and development evolve.

(c) Design input. Each manufacturer shall establish and maintain procedures to ensure that the design requirements relating to a device are appropriate and address the intended use of the device, including the needs of the user and patient. The procedures shall include a mechanism for addressing incomplete, ambiguous, or conflicting requirements. The design input requirements shall be documented and shall be reviewed and approved by a designated individual. The approval, including the date and signature of the individual(s) approving the requirements, shall be documented.

(d) Design output. Each manufacturer shall establish and maintain procedures for defining and documenting design output in terms that allow an adequate evaluation of conformance to design input requirements. Design output procedures shall contain or make reference to acceptance criteria, and shall ensure that those design outputs that are essential for the proper functioning of the device are identified. Design output shall be documented, reviewed, and approved before release. The approval, including the date and signature of the individual(s) approving the output, shall be documented.

(e) Design review. Each manufacturer shall establish and maintain procedures to ensure that formal documented reviews of the design results are planned and conducted at appropriate stages of the device's design development. The procedures shall ensure that participants at each design review include representatives of all functions concerned with the design stage being reviewed and an individual(s) who does not have direct responsibility for the design stage being reviewed, as well as any specialists needed. The results of a design review, including identification of the design, the date, and the individual(s)

performing the review, shall be documented in the design history file (the DHF).

(f) Design verification(s). Each manufacturer shall establish and maintain procedures for verifying the device design. Design verification shall confirm that the design outputs meet the design input requirements. The results of the design verification, including identification of the design, method(s), the date and the individual(s) performing the verification, shall be documented in the Design History File.

(g) Design validation. Each manufacturer shall establish and maintain procedures for validating the device product design. Design validation(s) shall be performed under defined operating conditions on initial production units, lots, or batches, or their equivalents. Design validation shall ensure that devices conform to defined user needs and intended uses and shall include testing of production units under actual or simulated use conditions. Design validation shall include software validation and risk analysis, where appropriate. The results of the design validation, including identification of the design, method(s), the date, and the individual(s) performing the validation, shall be documented in the DHF.

(h) Design transfer. Each manufacturer shall establish and maintain procedures to ensure that the device design is correctly translated into production specifications.

(i) Design changes. Each manufacturer shall establish and maintain procedures for the identification, documentation and validation or where appropriate the verification, review, and approval of design changes before their implementation.

(j) Design history file: Each manufacturer shall establish and maintain a DHF for each type of device/product. The DHF shall contain or reference the records necessary to demonstrate that the design was developed in accordance with the approved design plan and the requirements of this part.

Referencehttps://www.accessdata.fda.gov/scripts/cdrh/cfdocs/cfcfr/CFRSearch.cfm? FR=820.30

Global Harmonisation Task Force

The Global Harmonisation Task Force (aka GHTF) was a voluntary group of international medical device regulatory professionals from competent authorities and the regulated industry.

The purpose of the GHTF was to encourage convergence in regulatory practices related to ensuring the safety, effectiveness /performance and quality of medical devices, promoting technological innovation and facilitating international trade, and the primary way in which this was accomplished was via the publication and dissemination of harmonised guidance documents on basic regulatory practices.

These documents, which were developed by five different GHTF Study Groups, can be adopted/implemented by member national regulatory authorities. The relationships between the work of each Study Group can be represented schematically.

The GHTF also served as an information exchange forum through which countries with medical device regulatory systems under development could benefit from the experience of those with existing systems and/or pattern their practices upon those of GHTF founding members.

International Medical Device Regulators Forum

The International Medical Device Regulators Forum (aka IMDRF) was conceived in February 2011 as a forum to discuss future directions in medical device regulatory harmonisation. It is a voluntary group of medical device regulators from around the world who have come together to build on the strong foundational work of the Global Harmonisation Task Force on Medical Devices (GHTF), and to accelerate international medical device regulatory harmonisation and convergence.

Design Controls and Medical Devices

Design controls are a collection of practices and procedures that are incorporated into the design and development (D&D) process for a regulated product such as a medical device.

As outlined in the introduction, design controls are required per FDA's Quality System Regulation, 21 CFR Part 820.30. They apply to a large variety of medical devices with varying levels of complexity and application (implants, delivery systems, fixation, transient use). The regulation itself does not describe in detail the practices that must be used, rather it works to establish a framework that manufacturers must use when developing and implementing design controls. This framework operates in the world of GxP—Good Engineering, Laboratory and Manufacturing Practices.

The manufacturing and design of medical devices is a diverse area which covers simple, single-use devices, over-the-counter devices and more complex devices used by professional medical practitioners. Based upon quality assurance principles and quality by design, the application of GMP and Good Engineering Practice (GEP) design controls provide a structure and clear path from user needs (intended use) to product delivery through a step-by-step standardised process.

Fixing design issues as soon as they arise in development reduces the cost of doing so at a later point and ensures the resultant design is appropriate for its intended use. Similarly, it's critical to identify gaps in the design or the methods used to demonstrate design verification and design outputs.

The formal review process (design control and design reviews) assists engineers and managers in engaging with decisions and understanding them better. It also ensures that when future changes are made, they are documented, controlled and reviewed adequately with proper consideration to the design inputs.

Design Control Benefits	
Intended Use	Intended use is documented and fit for purpose.
Alignment	The device meets customer needs and other regulatory and safety requirements. Design inputs meet design outputs.
Design for Manufacture	The device is suitable for manufacture with reference to the available technology and operating costs.
Consistency	Different products move through the same design and development process. Fosters consistency in the organisation.

ISO 13485:2016 Quality Management System-Requirements for Regulatory Purposes (Inclusive of Design Controls)

ISO 13485 Clause 7 specifies the requirements for the design and development of devices as part of the product realisation process. It should be noted that organisations can opt to exclude specific requirements of ISO 13485, in cases where product realisation is not applicable.

However, any such exclusion should be based on sound rationale with the technical case clearly documented and approved by stakeholders. An example of this may be where design and development activities are not conducted by the manufacturer e.g. contract manufacturers.

Clause 7 (product realisation) of ISO 13485:2019 details requirements for design and development controls. Clause 7 includes the following subparts:

Clause 7.1 Planning of product realisation
Clause 7.2 Customer-related processes
Clause 7.3 Design and development
Clause 7.4 Purchasing
Clause 7.5 Production and service provision
Clause 7.6 Control of measuring devices

Section 7.3 (Design and development) comprises:

Clause 7.3.1 Design and development planning
Clause 7.3.2 Design and development inputs
Clause 7.3.3 Design and development outputs
Clause 7.3.4 Design and development review
Clause7.3.5 Design and development verification
Clause 7.3.6 Design and development validation
Clause 7.3.7 Control of design and development changes

Definitions

Change Management System: a management process where changes to the product design (labelling, packaging functionality, performance, safety etc.) or processes, facilities, utilities are assessed, planned and reviewed as part of a formal systematic process. In terms of design changes for products, the change management system must document if changes are designed to impact and determine actions and mitigations required to implement any changes effectively and safely.

Corrective Actions and Preventative Action (CAPA): when an unplanned or adverse event happens, corrective and preventative action can be implemented.

The Design and Development Plan (D&D Plan)

A D&D plan lists the activity required for the project, key milestones, design documents required, risk management documents required, regulatory and validation activity required. It may include roles and responsibilities for the functions of each team member. The plan should be approved by all functions or roles that form part of the project team. The DHF must include a design and development plan and any project schedule.

Design Review: a process of evaluating the design requirements against the ability of it to deliver the intended device.

Design History File (DHF): an approved list of records that describe the design history of a medical device. At the beginning of Design Control, a DHF should be created and then maintained. It should detail the design and development activities that relate to all aspects of the device such as the device itself, materials, components, labelling, packaging and production methods.

Design History Record (DHR): a record that contains the production history of a manufactured finished device. DHRs are issued for each lot or batch and provide traceability of materials and confirmation of testing and acceptance status.

Design Input: the physical, chemical, clinical, safety, regulatory, non-clinical, sterility, stability and performance requirements of a device that are the basis for the device design. Design inputs need to eventually trace to the design outputs and where tested provide verification and validation (V&V).

Design Output: the results of a design effort at each design phase and at the end of the total design effort. The finished design output is the basis for the device master record. The total finished design output consists of the device, its packaging and labelling, and the device master record.

Design Verification: confirmation by examination and provision of objective evidence that specified requirements have been fulfilled.

Design Transfer: DHF should include design transfer documentation showing that the device design was correctly translated into production specifications.

Design Validation: establishing by objective evidence that device or product specifications conform to user needs and intended use(s) defined in design documentation.

Device Master Record (DMR): a compilation of records containing the procedures and specification for a device. The contents of a DMR can contain local procedures such as SOPs and work instructions along with global or divisional specifications used to detail manufacturing processes, intermediate product or final product.

Design Phase Review(s): a documented, comprehensive, systematic examination of a design to evaluate the adequacy of the design requirements, the capability of the design to meet those requirements and to identify problems.

Intended Use: the use of a product, service or process as per the instructions for use or information provided by the manufacturer.

Independent Reviewer: A technically knowledgeable and experienced person without direct responsibility for the design under review.

Post-Launch Review: after the launch of a new product, a post-launch review is completed to monitor its safety and effectiveness and its risk and complaint performance.

Specification: specification means any requirement to which a product, process, service, or other activity must conform.

User Needs: knowing the intended use of a medical device allows the designer to then identify user needs. The device must be safe and effective for the user (patient or medical professional).

Validation: validation means confirmation by examination and provision of objective, documented evidence that the particular requirements for a specific intended use can be consistently fulfilled.

Design Reviews

The term "phased approach" is often used when describing the design control process. It simply means that a sequence of tasks needs to be completed, reviewed and approved during the development cycle of a product or medical device. Tasks can be grouped into phases or stages.

These different solutions then go on to be reviewed at the design selection process. At design selection, the project team must choose and justify a particular solution.

Design verification and validation ensures that the design is transferred to product launch and commercial supply. No change in the design intent also ensures that the device meets the user needs and intended uses (design inputs).

Design Planning Review

- Review ensures the intended use is documented.
- Design inputs are written and agreed early on in the design and development process.
- The overall approach to risk and risk management planning is commended.
- Timelines and resources to be reviewed.

Design Verification Review

- Ensures that the design outputs have fulfilled design inputs.
- Design inputs account for factors to ensure that the product remains safe.
- Design specifications meet design intent and are suitable for manufacturing requirements.

Design Validation

- Validation confirms the intended use is achieved and that the product is safe for use.
- Validation confirms that design inputs are fulfilled including regulatory requirements.

Design and Development Planning

It is the manufacturer's responsibility to establish and maintain plans that describe or reference the design and development activities and define responsibilities for implementation.

The plans should identify and describe the interaction with different groups or activities that are part of the design and development process.

The maintenance of plans to reflect an accurate state as the design and development progresses is also a key factor. The design and development planning is intended to be prospective in nature. It allows risks to be identified earlier and promotes timely delivery of projects.

Above all, it ensures that all key design and development tasks are addressed during the design and development process.

Design and Development Planning Objectives

• Describe the goals and objectives of the design and development project (i.e. what is to be developed).
• Definition and documentation of responsibilities.
• Identification of the major tasks and deliverables. Assign individual or organisational responsibilities.

Design Input

The aims of the Design Input Phase are to (1) define and document the user needs and the intended use of the medical device and (2) translate user needs and the intended use of the packaged device into design input requirements, e.g. engineering specifications and the product requirements specifications. The typical documents required when establishing design inputs include:

• The creation of a formal design description detailing the intended use, user requirements and design inputs. (Note: the design description must align with the design input requirements.)

• A design and development plan which provides an estimation of timelines, resources required, responsibilities, project risks and scope of the project.

• An initial risk assessment which contains the user, design and component risks to be mitigated.

• Design concepts and technology overview.

• Business case report addressing the market size and market opportunity.

Examples of design inputs include:

(a) **User Requirement:** the device must be sterile:
   a. Sterilisation via terminal sterilisation (e.g. ETO)
      i. The device material may not be compatible with ETO, therefore another method of sterilisation such as autoclaving via clean steam.

(b) **User Requirement:** Device is portable:
   a. Device must not be so heavy it cannot be easily carried.
      i. Quantify weight.

21 CFR Part 820.30(C) Design Input

- *Each manufacturer shall establish and maintain procedures to ensure that the design requirements relating to a device are appropriate and address the intended use of the device, including the needs of the user and patient.*
- *The procedures shall include a mechanism for addressing incomplete, ambiguous, or conflicting requirements.*
- *The design input requirements shall be documented and shall be reviewed and approved by designated individuals.*

Incomplete requirements can have a serious and costly effect on the design and ultimate success of a product. If essential design requirements are omitted in error or otherwise, the impact on quality or functionality may not be detected until validation. This presents an expensive problem that may not be easily rectified.

If design requirements are missed, a redesign may be necessary before a design can be released to production, and hence causing delays to the project. Furthermore, if modifications are required to tooling or process equipment, timelines can be impacted greatly.

However, the safety and quality of the product must be paramount.

Keeping one eye on the user requirements and intended use of the product is an important factor in avoiding gross design requirement failings.

Design input requirements must be comprehensive. This may be quite difficult for manufacturers who are implementing a system of design controls for the first time or for manufacturers who have various classes of products or complexity of products.

Design input requirements fall into three categories with most products having requirements within all three categories including:

(1) Functional requirements detailing the operation of the device.
(2) Performance requirements detailing the performance requirements or expectations of the device concerning the accuracy, speed of response times, battery life, device safety and reliability etc.
(3) Interface requirements specifying features of the device which are critical to compatibility with external systems such as the patient interface.

Design Inputs Checklist

- o   Device functions
- o   Physical characteristics
- o   Performance
- o   Safety
- o   Reliability
- o   Standards
- o   Regulatory requirements
- o   Human factors
- o   Labelling and packaging
- o   Maintenance (if required)
- o   Sterilisation
- o   Compatibility with other devices or products
- o   Environmental limits

Design Output

The purpose of the design selection (output) phase is to provide a range of design options and solutions with the relevant evidence to show the effectiveness of the same. Often proof of concept (POC) or proof of principle (POP) trials may be used to verify the effectiveness of solutions. There should be no contradictions or gaps between the documented inputs and outputs.

FDA 21 CFR Requirements—Design Output

21 CFR Part 820.30(D) Design Output

- *Each manufacturer shall establish and maintain procedures for defining and documenting design output in terms that allow an adequate evaluation of conformance to design input requirements.*
- *Design output procedures shall contain or make reference to acceptance criteria and shall ensure that those design outputs that are essential for the proper functioning of the device are identified.*
- *Design output shall be documented, reviewed, and approved before release.*
- *The approval, including the date and signature of the individual(s) approving the output, shall be documented.*

During this phase, product specifications (PS) and the device master record (DMR) are generated to define the design output. Planning for process validation and manufacturing begins during this phase often with the creation of a validation master plan (VMP). In any design, office or factory setting, a lot of data and paperwork are generated. Therefore, it is important to be able to make the distinction between what is a design output and what is not. The first way of identifying a design output is to verify if it is listed as a task, a deliverable or listed in the design and development plan. If this is the case, then it is classified as a design output. Furthermore, if it describes or defines a design feature, it can also be classed as a design output.

The quality system requirements for design output can be separated into two elements: design output should be expressed in terms that allow adequate assessment of conformance to design input requirements and should identify the characteristics of the design that are crucial to the safety and proper functioning of the device. This raises two fundamental issues for developers:

What constitutes design output?

As a general rule, an item is a design output if it is a work product or deliverable item of a design task listed in the design and development plan, and the item defines, describes, or elaborates an element of the design implementation.

Examples include block diagrams, flow charts, software high-level code, and system or subsystem design specifications.

The design output in one stage is often part of the design input in subsequent stages. Design output includes production specifications as well as descriptive materials which define and characterise the design.

Production Specifications

Production specifications draw upon many documents that are used to manufacture, test, inspect, install, maintain and service a device. They include (1) component and material specifications, (2) production and process specifications, (3) work instructions and SOPs, (4) quality plans, specifications and procedures, (4) labelling specifications, and (5) packaging specifications.

FDA 21 CFR Requirements- Design Review

FDA CFR Part 820.30(E) Design review

- *Each manufacturer shall establish and maintain procedures to ensure that formal documented reviews of the design results are planned and conducted at appropriate phases of the device's design development.*
- *The procedures shall ensure that participants at each design review include representatives of all functions concerned with the design phase being reviewed and an individual(s) who does not have direct responsibility for the design phase being reviewed, as well as any specialists needed.*
- *The results of a design review, including identification of the design, the date, and the individual(s) performing the review, shall be documented in the design history file (the DHF).*

Key goals of design review:

- provide feedback to designers on existing or emerging problems
- assess project progress
- provide confirmation that the project is ready to move on to the next phase of development

Many types of reviews occur during the course of developing a design.

A formal review of the design input requirements early in the development process is normally completed. The number of reviews depends upon the complexity of the device.

For a product involving multiple subsystems, an early design task is to allocate the design input requirements among the various subsystems. For example, in a microprocessor-based system, designers must decide which functions will be performed by hardware and which by software. In another case, tolerance build-up from several components may combine to create a clearance problem.

System designers must establish tolerance specifications for each component to meet the overall dimensional specification. In cases like these, a formal design review is a prudent step to ensure that all such system-level requirements have been allocated satisfactorily before engaging in the detailed design of each subsystem.

Many formal design reviews take the form of a meeting. At this meeting, the designer(s) may make presentations to explain the design implementation, and persons responsible for verification activities may present their findings to the reviewers. Reviewers may ask for clarification or additional information on any topic, and add their concerns to any raised by the presenters. This portion of the review is focused on finding problems, not resolving them. There are many approaches to conducting design review meetings. In simple cases, the technical assessor and reviewer may be the same person, often a project manager or engineering supervisor, and the review meeting is a simple affair in the manager's office. For more elaborate reviews, detailed written procedures are desirable to ensure that all pertinent topics are discussed, conclusions accurately recorded, and action items documented and tracked.

There is a dangerous tendency for design review meetings to become adversarial affairs. The reputation of the designers tends to be linked to the number of discrepancies found, causing the designers to become defensive, while the reviewers score points by finding weaknesses in the design.
The resulting contest can be counterproductive. An added complication is the presence of invited guests, often clinicians, who are expected to provide the user perspective. These reviewers are often very reluctant to ask probing questions, especially if they sense that they may become involved in a conflict where all the rules and relationships are not evident.

These difficulties can be avoided by stating the goals and ground rules for conducting the formal design review clearly at the outset.

While the designers are in the best position to explain the best features of the design, they are also most likely to be aware of the design's weaknesses. If the designers and reviewers are encouraged to work together to systematically explore problems and find solutions, the resultant design will be improved and all parties will benefit from the process. Participants must be encouraged to ask questions, avoid making assumptions, and think critically. The focus must be on the design, not the participants. Not all formal design reviews involve meetings. For extremely simple designs or design changes, it may be appropriate to specify a procedure in which review materials are distributed or circulated among the reviewers for independent assessment and approval. However, such a procedure negates the benefits of synergy and teamwork and should be considered only in cases where the design issues are limited in scope and well defined.

The reviewers consider concerns raised during the evaluation portion of the formal design review and decide on an appropriate disposition for each one. There is wide variation in the way companies implement decision-making processes. In some cases, the reviewers play an advisory role to the engineering manager or other company official, who directs the formal design review and ultimately selects a course of action. In other cases, the reviewers are given limited or broad authority to make decisions and commit resources to resolve problems. The approach used should be documented.

Design Inputs-Outputs and Verification (Matrix), IOV

The IOV matrix is a document that ensures all inputs are documented and associated with a design output and acceptance criteria. An example of a specific design input would include a product requiring sterility. The input requirement would be sterilisation (e.g. autoclaving). The design output along with the acceptance criteria would be "the product is sterile to a sterility assurance level of 1×10^{-6}.

Next is the design verification documentation or design validation documentation (as applicable) which should detail the report or document number related to the "sterility" testing.

Relationship Of Design Review to Verification and Validation

In practice, design review, verification, and validation overlap one another, and the relationship among them may be confusing. As a general rule, the sequence is verification, review, validation, review. In most cases, verification activities are completed before the design review, and the verification results are submitted to the reviewers along with the other design outputs to be reviewed. Alternatively, some verification activities may be treated as components of the design review, particularly if the verification activity is complex and requires multidisciplinary review. Similarly, validation typically involves a variety of activities, including a determination that the appropriate verifications and reviews have been completed. Thus, after the validation effort, a review is usually warranted to assure that the validation is complete and adequate.

Both clinical and non-clinical testing may be required to form the basis of verification activities when completed to determine what the design output specifications are. Typically, verification activities involve some scientific or chemical analysis and establish that the output specification is correct. Verification activities must be appropriate for the particular output that is being verified and documented.

Verification activities are completed via means of chemical/microbial analysis, inspection, measurement of an attribute, analysis or testing via other benchtop equipment.

Documenting Verification

The methods, plans, and protocols used for verifying design must be documented, reviewed and approved. All documents that provide evidence in support of verification results need to be added to the DHF.

Design Verification, Validation and Transfer Phase

To illustrate the concepts, consider a building design. In a typical scenario, the senior architect establishes the design input requirements and sketches the general appearance and construction of the building, but contractors typically elaborate and interpret the details into practical terms. Verification refers to the checking at each phase to ensure the output meets the design requirements. For example, if a device is designed to take both AC electrical power and a battery (DC power), the design engineer must verify that these are accounted for in the plans and production specifications.

FDA 21 CFR Requirements—Design Verification

FDA CFR Part 820.30(f) Design Verification

- *Each manufacturer shall establish and maintain procedures for verifying the device design.*
- *Design verification shall confirm that the design output meets the design input requirements.*
- *The results of the design verification, including identification of the design, method(s), the date, and the individual(s) performing the verification, shall be documented in the Design History File.*

The ultimate aim of design verification is to finalise design specification. Examples of verification activities include:

- Design failure modes and effects analysis (DFMEA)
- Fault tree analysis
- Package integrity tests
- Biocompatibility testing
- Bioburden testing of packed products
- Worst-case analysis—tolerance stacking of components

Design Validation

Design validation of the product is necessary to ensure the device meets the user requirements and intended use. Above all, it ensures the device operates reliably and safely. Process validation is required to confirm manufacturing specifications and the Device Master Record (DMR).

Validation is established via the documented evidence that the device as designed will perform and function as defined in the initial design input requirements and will meet defined intended uses as well as the needs of users/customer in the actual use environment.

FDA 21 CFR Requirements—Design Validation

FDA CFR 820.30(G) Design Validation

- *Each manufacturer shall establish and maintain procedures for validating the device design.*
- *Design validation shall be performed under defined operating conditions on initial production units, lots, batches, or their equivalents.*

- *Design validation shall ensure that devices conform to defined user needs, intended uses and shall include testing of production units under actual or simulated use conditions.*
- *Design validation shall include software validation and risk analysis, where appropriate.*
- *The results of the design validation, including identification of the design, method(s), the date, and the individual(s) performing the validation, shall be documented in the design history file.*

Verification examines design outputs at the different phases of the process while design validation confirms that all user needs are achieved even when subject to anticipated sources of variation such as materials, processing equipment, suppliers and so on.

Validation Review

Validation may expose deficiencies in the original assumptions concerning user needs and intended uses.

Many medical devices do not require clinical trials. However, all devices require a clinical evaluation and should be tested in the actual or simulated use environment as a part of validation.

This testing should involve devices which are manufactured using the same methods and procedures expected to be used for ongoing production. While testing is always a part of validation, additional validation methods are often used in conjunction with testing, including analysis and inspection methods, compilation of relevant scientific literature, provision of historical evidence that similar designs and/or materials are clinically safe, and full clinical investigations or clinical trials.

Some manufacturers have historically used their best assembly workers or skilled lab technicians to fabricate test articles, but this practice can obscure problems in the manufacturing process.

It may be beneficial to ask the best workers to evaluate and critique the manufacturing process by trying it out, but pilot production should simulate as closely as possible the actual manufacturing conditions.

Validation should also address product packaging and labelling. These components of the design may have significant human factors implications and may affect the product performance in unexpected ways. For example, packaging materials have been known to cause electrostatic discharge (ESD) failures in electronic devices.

If the unit under test is delivered to the test site in the test engineer's briefcase, the packaging problem may not become evident until after release to market.

Validation should include simulation of the expected environmental conditions, such as temperature, humidity, shock and vibration, corrosive atmospheres, etc.

For some classes of device, the environmental stresses encountered during shipment and installation far exceed those encountered during actual use and should be addressed during validation.

Design Transfer

The purpose of design transfer is to translate the design into the manufacturing setting and also finalise all deliverables for filing with regulatory agencies.

FDA 21 CFR Requirements—Design Transfer

FDA CFR Part 820.30(H) Design Transfer

- *Each manufacturer shall establish and maintain procedures to ensure that the device design is correctly translated into production specifications.*

As the design output is finalised, the design is transferred into production specifications (drawings, manufacturing, test, and inspection procedures). Production specifications must ensure that manufactured devices are consistently and reliably produced within product and process capabilities, meeting all quality requirements. No design team can anticipate all factors bearing on the success of the design, but procedures for design transfer should address at least the following basic elements:

First, the design and development procedures should include a qualitative assessment of the completeness and adequacy of the production specifications.

Second, the procedures should ensure that all documents and articles which constitute the production specifications are reviewed and approved.

Third, the procedures should ensure that only approved specifications are used to manufacture production devices.

The first item in the preceding list may be addressed during design transfer. The second and third elements are among the basic principles of document control and configuration management.

As long as the production specifications are traditional paper documents, there is ample information available to guide manufacturers in implementing suitable procedures.

When the production specifications include non-traditional means, flexibility and creativity may be needed to achieve comparable rigour. A post-launch review is required for each product within one year of the initial launch.

The purpose of the post-launch review is to confirm that no design or manufacturing changes are required and to document future product development activity. It also considers performance and patient safety. A mechanism should be established to track all change requests and change orders to ensure proper disposition.

Post-Transfer Design Change(s)

Design changes include revision to labelling such as primary packaging, secondary packaging and packaging inserts or changes to materials or product design. Each design change should be assessed for impact to design and safe function of the design but also the impact on design verifications and validations. Any new studies or verifications should be tracked and included in the Design History File for the product.

The impact on other documents such as risk management files should be assessed and documented. Design change control and management continues throughout the life of the product and should be governed by a company procedure.

Design Control Deliverables

Design and Development Plan: A design and development plan is an overarching document that describes the design and development, responsibilities, timelines and project scope, list and schedule of major tasks and the phase review details such as the timing and approval requirements.

Product Specification(s): The product specification is a design output document that is built throughout the project. Not all information will be final in the early phases, however, having an early draft will help focus minds and generate the right activity to define target dimensions, physical attributes and tolerances.

Stability Testing (verification): A document containing a summary of results, testing and analysis should be created and filed as part of the DHF.

Design Inputs/Outputs and Verification (Matrix), IOV

The IOV template is a document that ensures the design meets the user needs and they are detailed as Design Input(s), Output(s). Verification and validation are completed as applicable, with references to reports/studies provided.

Device Master Record: A DMR is an output document and should be available at the design transfer phase. It is a comprehensive list referencing all work instructions, test procedures, test specifications, manufacturing specifications and finished product specifications required to manufacture the product.

Test Method Validation: A list of all validated test methods (functional, analytical, physical etc.) should be available to file in the DHF.

Risk Management File: consisting of use and process FMEAs to ensure risk is reduced to as low as possible. The remaining risk or residual risk must include a risk-benefit analysis and must be acceptable. A risk management plan and risk report are requirements per ISO 14971. Design risk analysis should be maintained throughout the life cycle of the product to ensure it remains sage and reflective of the design intent.

Design History File: The DHF is a repository for all of the documentation generated as a result of the design control process. The DHF serves as a complete record of the design. It may be in electronic or physical format or a mixture of both.

Review and Inspection of Design Controls

1 *Select a single design project.*
   For the design project selected, verify that design control procedures that address the requirements of Section 820.30 of the regulation have been defined and documented.

2 *Review the design plan for the selected project to understand the layout of the design and development activities including assigned responsibilities and interfaces.*

3 *Confirm that design inputs were established.*

4 *Verify that the design outputs that are essential for the proper functioning of the device were identified.*

5 *Verify that the design outputs that are essential for the proper functioning of the device were identified.*

6 *Confirm that acceptance criteria were established before the performance of verification and validation activities.*

7 *Determine if design verification confirmed that design outputs met the design input requirements.*

8 *Confirm that design validation data show that the approved design met the predetermined user needs and intended uses.*

9 *Confirm that the completed design validation did not leave any unresolved discrepancies.*

10 *If the device contains software, confirm that the software was validated..*

11 *Confirm that risk analysis was performed.*

12 *Determine if design validation was accomplished using initial production devices or their equivalents.*

13 *Confirm that changes were controlled including validation or where appropriate verification.*

14 *Determine if design reviews were conducted.*

15 *Determine if the design was correctly transferred.*

Inspection and Review in detail (FDA Guidance)

1 For a particular design project or change control, verify that the design control procedures address the requirements of FDA 21 Section 820.30 of the regulation and have been defined and documented.

The scope of FDA CFR Section 820.30 Design Controls applies to the design of Class II and III medical devices, and a select group of Class I devices. In general, the regulation is very flexible in design controls and allows for medical device companies to establish design controls that make the best sense for their sub-industry and product type. However, the design and implementation of design controls should first and foremost consider the complexity of the device and associated risks. Software validation is included in FDA 21 CFR Section 820.30(g) Design Validation. If a device employs software, a review of the software's validation is also prudent while completing the assessment of the design control management system.

2 Review the design plan for the selected project to understand the layout of the design and development activities including assigned responsibilities and interfaces.

Written or electronic procedures are required by companies manufacturing medical devices. Procedures form the basis of the design control system and must be maintained and reviewed periodically. An inspection of Design control procedures should determine if the design input procedures include a mechanism for addressing incomplete, ambiguous, or conflicting requirements. Design output procedures ensure that critical design outputs for the proper functioning of the device are identified; and the design review procedure ensures that each design review includes an individual(s) who does not have direct responsibility for the design stage being reviewed.

3   Confirm that design inputs were established.

Research and development studies do not require design controls to be applied, however, many firms still employ some level of change control, management oversight and Good Engineering Practice. Once a decision is made to develop a particular design, a design plan must be established. Design control can begin at this point but *must* begin prior to the first set of design inputs being established. Plans must define responsibility for implementation of the design and development activities and identify and describe the relationships with different groups or activities.

4   Verify that the design outputs that are essential for the proper functioning of the device were identified.

Inputs are the requirements of a device based on the intended use. Sources of design inputs include the voice of the consumer, regulations, standards (ISO, ASTM) etc. Review the sources used to develop inputs. The design inputs should cover all relevant aspects such as *intended use, risk, performance characteristics, biocompatibility, compatibility, human factors, sterility* and *the intended environment of use.*

5   Verify that the design outputs that are essential for the proper functioning of the device were identified.

Design outputs are the work products or deliverables of a design stage. Examples include diagrams, drawings, specifications and procedures. The outputs from one stage may become inputs to the next stage. The total finished design output consists of the device, its packaging and labelling, and the device master record. Important linkages to consider are Sections 820.80 Receiving, In-Process, And Finished Device Acceptance, 820.120 Device Labelling, and 820.130 Device Packaging. Design projects can produce a large volume of records. Not all of the records generated during the project are design outputs and as such do not need to be retained in the design history file. Only approved outputs need to be retained.

Outputs must be comprehensive enough to characterise the device design to allow for verification and validation. Also, design outputs which are essential for the proper functioning of the device must be identified. Typically a risk analysis tool such as FTA or FMEA is used to determine essential outputs. For the selected project, verify that essential outputs have been identified. In addition, review the firm's process for determining how the essential outputs were identified and determine if it was done in accordance with their design output procedures.

Important linkages to consider are Sections 820.50 Purchasing Controls, and 820.100 Corrective and Preventive Action.

Verification and validation activities should be predictive rather than empiric. Acceptance criteria must be stated up front. Review the documentation associated with a sample of verification activities and a sample of validation activities as determined using the sampling tables. If possible, select activities that are associated with outputs identified as essential to the proper functioning of the device. Confirm that acceptance criteria were established prior to the performance of verification or validation activity.

6   Confirm that acceptance criteria were established prior to the performance of verification and validation activities.

Design verification activities are performed to provide objective evidence that design output meets the design input requirements. Verification activities include tests, inspections, analyses, measurements, or demonstrations. Activities should be explicit and thorough in their execution. It is the firm's responsibility to select and apply appropriate verification techniques. Complex designs can require more and different types of verification activities than simple designs. Any approach selected by the firm, as long as it establishes conformance of the output to the input, is an acceptable means of verifying the design for that requirement.

Review the documentation of the verification activities associated with a sample of inputs and outputs as determined using the sampling tables. If possible, select activities that are associated with outputs identified as essential to the proper functioning of the device. Confirm that design outputs met design input requirements.

1   **Determine if design verification confirmed that design outputs met the design input requirements.**

Design validation is performed to provide objective evidence that device specifications (outputs) conform to user needs and intended use(s). Design validation must be completed before commercial distribution of the device.

Design validation involves the performance of clinical evaluations and includes testing under actual or simulated use conditions. Clinical evaluations can include clinical investigations or clinical trials, but they may also involve other activities. These may include evaluations in clinical or non-clinical settings, provision of historical evidence that similar designs are clinically safe, or a review of scientific literature. Validation activities must address the needs of all relevant parties (i.e. patient, health care worker, etc.) and be performed for each intended use. Validation activities should address the design outputs of labelling and packaging. These outputs may have human factor implications, and may adversely affect the device and its use. If possible, review the evaluations (clinical or other activities) performed to assist in validating the device design.

2   Confirm that design validation data show that the approved design met the predetermined user needs and intended uses.

Design validation may detect discrepancies between the device specifications (outputs) and the needs of the user or intended use(s) of the device. All discrepancies must be addressed and resolved by the firm. This can be accomplished through a change in design output or a change in user need or intended use.

3   Confirm that the completed design validation did not leave any unresolved discrepancies.

As previously noted, design validation includes the requirement for software validation. If the selected device is software controlled then its software must be validated.

4   If the device contains software, confirm that the software was validated.

As previously noted, a risk analysis must be completed in design validation.

5   Confirm that risk analysis was performed.

Initial production units, lots, or batches, or their equivalents are to be used in design validation. Confirm that such production devices or their equivalents were used by reviewing the design validation documentation. If production devices were not used, the firm must demonstrate equivalency to production devices. When the so-called "equivalent" devices are used in design validation the manufacturer must document in detail how the device was manufactured, and how the manufacturing is similar and possibly different from initial production. Where there are differences, the manufacturer must justify why design validation results are valid for production units, lots or batches. The regulation is flexible and it does allow for the use of equivalent devices, but the burden is on the manufacturer to document that the units were indeed equivalent.

Process validation may be conducted concurrently with design validation. Production devices used in design validation may have been manufactured in a production run during process validation.

6   Determine if design validation was accomplished using initial production devices or their equivalents.

Change control is not a new requirement. The 1978 GMP regulation Section 820.100(a)(2) required approval of changes made to specifications after final design transfer (post-production changes). The Quality System regulation clarified and relocated the requirement into Section 820.30(i). It expanded the requirement to include changes made during the design process (preproduction changes).

The documentation and control of design changes begin when the initial design inputs are approved and continues for the life of the product. Examples of the application of change control include: changes made to approved inputs or outputs such as to correct design deficiencies identified in the verification and validation activities; labelling changes; changes which enhance the device's capabilities or the capabilities of the process; and changes resulting from customer complaints.

Product development is inherently an evolutionary process. While change is a healthy and necessary part of product development, quality can be ensured only if change is controlled and documented in the development process, as well as in the production process.

The degree of design change control is dependent on the significance of the change and the risk presented by the device. Manufacturers may use their routine post-production change control procedure for preproduction design changes. However, most post-production change control procedures may be too restrictive and stifle the development process. Firms may use a separate and less stringent change control procedure for preproduction design changes.

Post-production design changes require the firm to loop back into the design controls of Section 820.30 of the regulation. This does not mean that post-production changes have to go back to the R&D Department for processing. This track is dependent on what the firm specifies in its change procedure. It is acceptable for the manufacturing department to process the entire design change and to implement the controls of Section 820.30. The design change control section is linked to Section 820.70(b) Production and Process Changes Of The Regulation.

All design changes must be verified. Design changes must also be validated unless the performance of only verification can be justified and documented by the firm. Where a design change cannot be verified by subsequent inspection and test, it must be validated. For example, a change in the intended use of the device will require validation. However, if a firm was making a design change in the material used in the device, then verification through analysis may only be required. The burden is on the firm to justify and document why verification only is appropriate in place of validation.

Review preproduction and a post-production design change.

13 Confirm that changes were controlled including validation or where appropriate verification

Formal design reviews are planned and typically conducted at the end of each design stage or phase, or after completion of project milestones. The number of reviews is dependent on the complexity of the design. A single review may be appropriate at the conclusion of the design project for a simple design or a minor change to an existing product. Multiple reviews are typically conducted for projects involving subsystems or complex designs.

Design reviews should provide feedback to designers on existing or emerging problems, assess the progress of the design, and confirm the design is ready to move to the next phase of development. Reviews should focus on the ability to produce the design and whether the design meets the input requirements. The design review process should account for risk analysis and change control where relevant.

Full convened meetings with an agenda, minutes, etc. need not take place for all design reviews. Meetings may not be necessary for reviews involving simple designs or minor changes. In these cases, desk reviews and sign-offs by the various organisational components including an individual not having direct responsibility for the design stage being reviewed may be appropriate. However, such reviews must still be documented and covered by defined and documented procedures.

Review the records of one design review and confirm that the review included an individual without direct responsibility for the design stage being reviewed. Also, confirm that outstanding action items are being resolved or have been resolved.

While in some respects it is a separate area of expertise, risk management has an integral role in design control and should be factored into the design and development stage of the project and throughout the life cycle of the product.

Identification of the user needs and intended use and application of the device is recognised as the first step in the risk assessment process. At the design input phase and design selection phase, risk assessments should be in a mature state.

Potential risks relating to the design of the product. Unacceptable risks can be dealt with through revisiting the design or introducing controls or mitigations to reduce the risks to acceptable levels.

Following on from the design and development phase, the design verification, validation and transfer phases, or the clinical readiness phase, risk management activities and acceptability of the residual risk become the focus and must be approved indicating acceptability. This is often referred to as communicated risk.

Internal Requirements (Company requirements)

In order to apply a risk management strategy, a procedure or SOP on risk management is typically available within manufacturing companies. This should clearly describe the risk management process and the various risk assessment tools, their application and guidance on how to complete them. The content of any risk management procedure or SOP should align with ISO 14971:2007.

14 Determine if design reviews were conducted

Formal design reviews are planned and typically conducted at the end of each design stage or phase, or after completion of project milestones. The number of reviews is dependent on the complexity of the design. A single review may be appropriate at the conclusion of the design project for a simple design or a minor change to an existing product. Multiple reviews are typically conducted for projects involving subsystems or complex designs.

Design reviews should provide feedback to designers on existing or emerging problems, assess the progress of the design, and confirm the design is ready to move to the next phase of development. Reviews should focus on the ability to produce the design and whether the design meets the input requirements.

The design review process should account for risk analysis and change control where relevant.

Fully convened meetings with an agenda, minutes, etc. need not take place for all design reviews. Meetings may not be necessary for reviews involving simple designs or minor changes. In these cases, desk reviews and sign-offs by the various organisational components including an individual not having direct responsibility for the design stage being reviewed may be appropriate. However, such reviews must still be documented and covered by defined and documented procedures.

Review the records of one design review and confirm that the review included an individual without direct responsibility for the design stage being reviewed. Also, confirm that outstanding action items are being resolved or have been resolved.

15 Determine if the design was correctly transferred

The transfer process must be a part of the design plan. It is not uncommon for the design to be transferred in phases. Production specifications typically consist of written documents such as assembly drawings, inspection and test specifications and manufacturing instructions. However, they can also consist of electronic records, training materials such as videotapes or pictures, and manufacturing jigs and moulds.

Review how the design was transferred into production specifications. Review the device master record. Sample the significant elements of the device master record using the sampling tables and compare these with the approved design outputs. These elements may be chosen based on the firm's previously identified essential requirements and risk analysis.

Part II Risk Management

Introduction

Risk management is the systematic application of risk management policies and procedures that are intended to identify, analyse, control and monitor risk and its impact on a product or patient.

An example of this is an exposure control system for a general-purpose x-ray system. The control function was allocated to software. Late in the development process, risk analysis of the system uncovered several failure modes that could result in overexposure to the patient. Because the problem was not identified until the design was near completion, an expensive, independent, back-up timer had to be added to monitor exposure times.

Risk Control

Where risks are identified as unacceptable, risk control measures must be determined to reduce the risk prior to the process or system being implemented. Several actions can be taken to further reduce risk including (1) changing the design to reduce risk, introducing protective measures in the device or the manufacturing process, (3) inserting a warning statement into the instructions for use (IFU).

Risks scored as "investigate further risk reduction" should be examined to determine whether it is practicable to reduce the risk further. The risk should be reduced to as low as is reasonably practicable, (aka ALARP) taking into account the benefits of accepting the risk and the practicability of implementation. If risks classed as "investigate further risk reduction" are already at ALARP, no further risk reduction is necessary.

Residual Risk Evaluation

After risk control measures are applied, a new risk assessment will be carried out to determine residual risks. If the residual risk is not judged acceptable then further risk control measures will be applied.

If the residual risk is not judged acceptable and further risk control is not practicable then the team may perform a risk/benefit analysis by evaluating data and literature on the medical benefits of the intended use to determine if they outweigh the risk. If this evidence does not support the conclusion that the medical benefits outweigh the residual risk, then the risk remains unacceptable. This analysis should be recorded and approved by both the risk management team and senior site management.

Residual risks are evaluated by the same method and with the same criteria for risk acceptability as the initial risks. The residual risk is either acceptable or unacceptable.

IF UNACCEPTABLE—further risk control options should be investigated. If further risk control is not practicable, a benefit-risk analysis may be performed.

Benefit-Risk Analysis

A benefit-risk analysis for those risks that are not judged acceptable using the criteria established in the risk management plan and for which further risk control is not practicable. The benefit-risk analysis is used to determine if the residual risk is outweighed by the expected benefits of the intended use of the medical device.

Residual Risk Evaluation

Residual risks are evaluated by the same method and with the same criteria for risk acceptability as the initial risks. The residual risk is either acceptable or unacceptable. IF UNACCEPTABLE—further risk control options should be investigated. If further risk control is not practicable, a benefit-risk analysis may be performed.

ISO 14971: 2009— Characteristics—Annexe C

Annexee C contains several questions that can be used to identify medical device characteristics that could impact upon safety:

1)What is the intended use and how is the medical device to be used?

2)Is the medical device intended to be implanted?

3)Is the medical device intended to be in contact with the patient or other persons?

4)What materials or components are utilised in the medical device or are used with, or are in contact with, the medical device?

ISO 14971:2009— Annexee E

Refer to EN ISO 14971:2009 Annexee E - Examples of Hazards, Foreseeable Sequences Of Events and Hazardous Situations.

Examples of hazards, foreseeable sequences of events and hazardous situations:

Examples of energy hazards

Electromagnetic energy
Line voltage
Leakage current
- enclosure leakage current
- earth leakage current
- patient leakage current
Electric fields
Magnetic fields
Radiation energy
Ionising radiation
Non-ionising radiation
Thermal energy
High temperature
Low temperature
Mechanical energy
Gravity

Examples of biological and chemical hazards

Bacteria
Viruses
Other agents (e.g. prions)
Re- or cross-infection
Chemical

Exposure of airway, tissues, environment or property, e.g. to foreign materials:
- acids or alkalis
- residues
- contaminates
- additives or processing aids
- cleaning, disinfecting or testing agents
- degradation products
- medical gases
- anaesthetic products

Biocompatibility
Toxicity of chemical constituents

Example of operational hazards

Function
Incorrect or inappropriate output or functionality
Incorrect measurement
Erroneous data transfer
Loss or deterioration of function

Use error
Attentional failure
Memory failure
Rule-based failure
Knowledge-based failure
Routine violation

Examples of information hazards

Labelling
Incomplete instructions for use
Inadequate description of performance characteristics
Inadequate specification of intended use
Inadequate disclosure of limitations

Operating instructions
Inadequate specification of accessories to be used with the medical device
Inadequate specification of pre-use checks

Over-complicated operating instructions

Warnings
Of side effects
Of hazards likely with re-use of single-use medical devices

Examples of initiating events and circumstances

Incomplete requirements
Inadequate specification of:
- design parameters
- operating parameters
- performance requirements
- in-service requirements (e.g. maintenance, reprocessing)

end of life

Manufacturing processes
Insufficient control of changes to manufacturing processes
Insufficient control of materials/materials compatibility
information
Insufficient control of manufacturing processes
Insufficient control of subcontractors

Transport and storage
Inadequate packaging
Contamination or deterioration

Inappropriate environmental conditions

Environmental factors
Physical (e.g. heat, pressure, time)
Chemical (e.g. corrosions, degradation, contamination)
Electromagnetic fields (e.g. susceptibility to electromagnetic
disturbance)
Inadequate supply of power

Inadequate supply of coolant

Cleaning, disinfection and sterilisation

Lack of, or inadequate specification for, validated procedures for cleaning, disinfection and sterilisation

Inadequate conduct of cleaning, disinfection and sterilisation

Disposal and scrapping

No information or inadequate information provided

Use error

Formulation

Biodegradation
Biocompatibility
No information or inadequate specification provided
Inadequate warning of hazards associated with incorrect formulations

Use error

Human factors

Potential for use errors triggered by design flaws, such as
- confusing or missing instructions for use
- complex or confusing control system
- ambiguous or unclear device state
- ambiguous or unclear presentation of settings, measurements or other information
- misinterpretation of results
- insufficient visibility, audibility or tactility
- poor mapping of controls to actions, or of displayed information to actual state
- controversial modes or mapping as compared to existing equipment
- use by unskilled/untrained personnel
- insufficient warning of side effects
- inadequate warning of hazards associated with re-use of single-use medical devices
- incorrect measurement and other metrological aspects

- incompatibility with consumables/accessories/other medical devices

slips, lapses and mistakes

The Quality System and Design Controls

In addition to procedures and work instructions necessary for the implementation of design controls, policies and procedures may also be needed for other determinants of device quality that should be considered during the design process. The need for policies and procedures for these factors is dependent upon the types of devices manufactured by a company and the risks associated with their use. Management with executive responsibility has the responsibility for determining what is needed.

Example of topics for which policies and procedures may be appropriate are:

Risk management	Configuration management
Device reliability	Compliance with regulatory requirements
Device durability	Device evaluation
Device maintainability	Clinical evaluations
Device serviceability	Document controls
Human factors engineering	Use of consultants
Software engineering	Use of subcontractors
Use of standards	Use of company historical data

Risk Classification

With the exception of in vitro diagnostic medical devices and active implantable medical devices, medical devices are allocated to risk classes that are mainly based on the potential damage that can be caused by an error/malfunction of the medical device. These risk classes range from Class I (low risk) and IIa and IIb to Class III (high risk). Class I products are additionally subdivided according to whether they require sterilisation (Is) or include a measuring function (Im) which is relevant for the further conformity assessment procedure. The classification is based on the rules laid down in Annexe IX of Council Directive 93/42/EEC. The following rules are most suitable for the classification of stand-alone software.

Rule 9

"All active therapeutic devices intended to administer or exchange energy are in Class IIa unless their characteristics are such that they may administer or exchange energy to or from the human body in a potentially hazardous way, taking account of the nature, the density and site of application of the energy, in which case they   are   in   Class   IIb.
All active devices intended to control or monitor the performance of active therapeutic devices in Class IIb, or intended directly to influence the performance of such devices are in Class IIb."

Rule 10

"Active devices intended for diagnosis are in Class IIa,

- if they are intended to supply energy which will be absorbed by the human body, except for devices used to illuminate the patient's body, in the visible spectrum;

- if they are intended to image in vivo distribution of radiopharmaceuticals;

- if they are intended to allow direct diagnosis or monitoring of vital physiological processes, unless they are specifically intended for monitoring of vital physiological parameters, where the nature of variations is such that it could result in immediate danger to the patient, for instance, variations in cardiac performance, respiration, activity of CNS in which case they are in Class IIb.

- Active devices intended to emit ionising radiation and intended for diagnostic and therapeutic interventional radiology including devices which control or monitor such devices, or which directly influence their performance, are in Class IIb."

Rule 12

"All other active devices are in Class I."

Rule 14

"All devices used for contraception or the prevention of the transmission of sexually transmitted diseases are in Class IIb, ..."

The following definitions in accordance with Annexe IX Section I No. 1 of Council Directive 93/42/EEC are to be observed:

- **Stand-alone software**

  Stand-alone software is considered to be an active medical device.

- **Active therapeutic device**

"Any active medical device, whether used alone or in combination with other medical devices, to support, modify, replace or restore biological functions or structures with a view to treatment or alleviation of an illness, injury or handicap."

- **Active device for diagnosis**

"Any active medical device, whether used alone or in combination with other medical devices, to supply information for detecting, diagnosing, monitoring or treating physiological conditions, states of health, illnesses or congenital deformities."

The aforementioned rules show that medical apps on smartphones and tablets will mostly be classified in risk Class I in accordance with Rule 12. If the medical devices are intended for diagnosis or monitoring of vital functions (e.g. cardiac functions), Classes IIa or IIb can also be considered.

Depending on the risk class there are different requirements for conducting a conformity assessment procedure as the prerequisite for affixing the CE marking and for correct marketing within the European Economic Area.

Thus, the manufacturer can perform a conformity assessment e.g. for Class I devices without involvement of a notified body; for all other risk classes (also in the case of Class I devices that require sterilisation or include a measuring function) it is mandatory to involve a notified body. If a stand-alone software or app is placed on the market as a medical device it is subject to the same regulations as all other medical devices.

Part III: MDR 2017/745

Regulatory Framework

The new European regulations on medical devices and in vitro medical devices were adopted on 05 April 2017 and came into force on 25th May 2017. Both these two new regulations replace and repeal Council Directives 90/385/EEC, 93/42/EEC Directive 98/79/EC and Commission Decision 2010/227/EU. Although adopted and in force, the new rules only applied after a three-year transitional period, whereby regulations entered into force in April 2020 for medical devices and for five years after entry into force (April 2022) for the regulation on in vitro diagnostic medical devices. The core goal of the new MDR rules and regulations is aimed at establishing a modern and robust EU legislative framework to ensure better patient safety and quality from manufacturers.

A seismic scandal concerning fraudulent production of PIP silicone breast implants highlighted weaknesses in the legal system in place at the time and damaged the confidence of patients, consumers and healthcare professionals in the safety of medical devices.

Such problems should not occur again and the safety of all medical devices available in the EU has to be strengthened. Moreover, revision of the legislation was necessary to consolidate the role of the EU as a global leader in the sector over the long-term and to take into account all technological and scientific developments in the sector.

Problems with diverging interpretation of the current directives as well as the incident concerningThe new regulations will ensure:

a consistently high level of health and safety protection for EU citizens using these products the free and fair trade of the products throughout the EU

that EU legislation is adapted to the significant technological and scientific progress occurring in this sector over the last 20 years

MDR Implementation

From 26 November 2017, conformity assessment bodies were ineligible to apply for designation as notified bodies under Regulations (EU) 2017/745 and 2017/746.

Guidance documents and forms are provided by the *MDCG*. A joint assessment conducted onsite is also a requirement for designation of a notified body.

This **rolling plan** contains the list of essential implementing acts and actions for the transitional period as well as information on expected timelines and state-of-play. Its two main sections are implementing acts and other actions/initiatives. The rolling plan will be reviewed quarterly to provide operators with the latest information.

Use this document together with the **'MDR/IVDR roadmap'**, produced by the Competent Authorities for Medical Devices Project (CAMD) and the Commission. The roadmap is more comprehensive. It gives an overview of all the Commission's and national competent authorities' expected initiatives (including guidance) during the transitional period.

Medical Device Coordination Group

The Medical Device Coordination Group (MDCG) is an expert group established by Regulation, (EU) 2017/745 on medical devices and Regulation (EU) 2017/746 on in vitro diagnostic medical devices. Members are experts representing competent authorities in all EU countries. The MDCG provides advice and expertise, assisting the Commission/EU in implementation of both regulations.

Article 103 (1) of Regulation (EU)2017/7451 establishes the Medical Device Coordination Group (MDCG). Per Article 103(9) of Regulation (EU) 2017/745 and Article 98 of Regulation (EU) 2017/7462, the MDCG group carries out the tasks conferred on it under both Regulations. Article 105 of Regulation (EU) 2017/745 and Article 99 of Regulation (EU) 2017/746 define general tasks of the MDCG. Specific tasks and roles of the MDCG are laid down in various provisions of the Regulations. The terms of reference document cover the following topics:

(Official EU Reference website)
http://ec.europa.eu/transparency/regexpert/index.cfm?do=group Detail.groupDetailDoc&id=37277&no=1

MDCG Rules of Procedure

Having regard to the standard rules of procedure of expert groups, the following rules of procedure have been adopted:

For the manufacturer or authorised representative, the terms of reference and rules of procedure do not impact directly on the application of the new MDR rules. However, they are included here for general information, reference purposes and completeness.

The MDCG is currently made up of 11 distinct **working groups**:

1. Notified Bodies Oversight, (NBO)
2. Standards
3. Clinical Investigation and Evaluation, (CIE)
4. Post-Market Surveillance and Vigilance (PMSV)
5. Market Surveillance
6. Borderline and Classification (B&C)

7. New Technologies
8. Eudamed – see the register of Expert Groups under the code E01309
9. Unique Device Identification, (UDI)
10. International Matters
11. In vitro diagnostic medical devices, (IVD)

Notified Bodies Oversight (NBO)—Terms of reference

The following information is available via the European Union

NBO provides assistance to the MDCG on issues relating to notified bodies and conformity assessments, with the aim of consistent, effective and harmonised application and implementation of Regulation (EU) 2017/745 on medical devices (MDR) and Regulation (EU) 2017/746 on in-vitro diagnostic medical devices (IVDR). NBO provides a forum for sharing of experience and coordination of administrative practice among authorities responsible for notified bodies (the designating authorities), in accordance with Articles 48(1) MDR / 44(1) IVDR. NBO prepares draft best practice documents and model forms relating to the activities of designating authorities, notified bodies and their conformity assessment activities, for endorsement of the MDCG. NBO advises the Commission, at its request, on matters concerning the Coordination Group of Notified Bodies, as referred to in Articles 49 MDR / 45 IVDR.

2. Standards—Terms of reference

The Working Group on Standards provides assistance to the MDCG on issues relating to standardisation in the field of medical devices, in particular harmonised standards referred to in Article 8 of Regulation (EU) 2017/745 on medical devices (MDR) and Article 8 of Regulation (EU) 2017/746 on in-vitro diagnostic medical devices (IVDR). In particular, the group deals with harmonised standards where problems or safety-related issues are identified and makes proposals for solutions. In addition, it provides advice to the MDCG and other working groups on the availability of harmonised standards in the context of preparation of common specifications referred to in Articles 9 MDR / 9 IVDR. The group supports establishing a coordinated and more effective cooperation with the European and international standardisation organisations, in particular in the context of the International Medical Device Regulators Forum (IMDRF). It contributes to the development of proposals for standardisation requests to the European Standardisation Organisations.

3. Clinical Investigation and Evaluation (CIE)—Terms of reference

CIE assists the MDCG on issues relating to clinical investigation and evaluation of medical devices in accordance with Regulation (EU) 2017/745 (MDR). In the field of its activities, the group prepares draft guidance, for endorsement by the MDCG. In addition, CIE develops proposals for common specifications in respect of the clinical investigation, evaluation and post-market clinical follow-up, as referred to in Article 9 MDR

4. Post-Market Surveillance and Vigilance (PMSV)—Terms of reference

PMSV assists the MDCG on issues related to post-market surveillance, incident reporting and vigilance, with the aim of effective and harmonised application and implementation of Regulation (EU) 2017/745 on medical devices (MDR) and Regulation (EU) 2017/746 on in-vitro diagnostic medical devices (IVDR). It prepares draft technical guidance and forms for use, for endorsement of the MDCG. It also assists the MDCG in coordinating the activities of the competent authorities of Member States in the field of vigilance. PMSV provides a forum for sharing of information and experience, discussing actual incident cases, reviewing current reporting practices and discussion and sharing of suspected safety signals and trends detected from the relevant data sources. It provides advice on matters related to manufacturers' post-market surveillance responsibilities, including use of terminologies, post-market clinical follow-up (PMCF)/ post-market performance follow-up (PMPF), device registries, real-world data and other data sources, including the existing pharmacovigilance systems. PMSV contributes to the development of measures aimed to improve post-market surveillance and the reporting behaviour of the relevant actors. Where appropriate, it contributes to international guidance and practice in this area e.g. IMDRF, WHO, etc

PMSV operates in accordance with the terms and rules applicable to the MDCG unless specified otherwise in these Terms of Reference. PMSV shall be chaired by a representative of the Commission. Where appropriate, it may be co-chaired by a member of the working group. PMSV shall report to the MDCG. The meetings are convened by the Chair. PMSV shall meet either in physical meetings or for audio- or videoconferences. Physical meetings of PMSV take place at least twice a year. A teleconference takes place once a month. Minutes on the discussion on each point on the agenda and on the positions delivered by the group shall be meaningful and complete. PMSV coordinates its activities with other MDCG working groups as appropriate.

5. Market Surveillance—Terms of reference

The Working Group on Market Surveillance assists the MDCG in its endeavour to coordinate market surveillance. This includes the development and maintenance of a framework for a European market surveillance programme, to achieve efficiency and harmonisation of market surveillance in the Union, in accordance with Article 93 of Regulation (EU) 2017/745 on medical devices (MDR) and Article 88 of Regulation (EU) 2017/746 on in-vitro diagnostic medical devices (IVDR). The group deals, among others, with an analysis of: (i) the application and implementation of the general safety and performance requirements, set out in Annexe I of the MDR / Annexee I of the IVDR; (ii) general obligations of economic operators laid down in Chapter II of the MDR / Chapter II of the IVDR; (iii) obligations of economic operators and conformity assessment with regard to products that do not require the involvement of notified bodies. In the field of its activities, the group prepares draft guidance, for endorsement of the MDCG.

6. Borderline and Classification (B&C)—Terms of reference

The Working Group on Borderline and Classification provides assistance to the MDCG on issues related to: (i) qualification of a product as a medical device / an accessory for a medical device under Regulation (EU) 2017/745 (MDR), and in-vitro diagnostic medical device / an accessory for an in-vitro diagnostic medical device under Regulation (EU) 2017/746 (IVDR); (ii) qualification of products without an intended medical purpose in accordance with Annexe XVI MDR; (iii) classification of medical devices in accordance with Annexe VIII MDR and classification of in-vitro diagnostic medical devices in accordance with Annexe VIII IVDR. The group prepares draft guidance on qualification and classification, for endorsement by the MDCG. It provides a forum for an exchange of information and coordination of national practices as regards qualification and classification of devices, in accordance with the consultation mechanism – the so-called "Helsinki Procedure". The group prepares a compendium of qualification and classification entries following from the application of the "Helsinki Procedure" in the form of a "Manual on Borderline and Classification". 2. Membership Members/observers to the group are experts appointed by Member States and third countries participating in the MDCG. Member States / third countries may appoint alternates. Appointments are not time-limited. Any changes in the appointment shall be notified to the Commission without delay. Stakeholders may participate in the open sessions of the group either in the capacity of observers or following ad hoc invitations, in accordance with the Rules of Procedure of the MDCG.

7. New Technologies—Terms of reference

The Working Group on New Technologies provides assistance to the MDCG on issues related to the application of new and emerging technologies to medical devices under Regulation (EU) 2017/745 (MDR) and in-vitro diagnostic medical device under Regulation (EU) 2017/746 (IVDR), including software, apps and cybersecurity. In particular, the group analyses the adequacy of the existing regulatory framework in relation to those issues and

technologies and, where challenges are identified, it provides recommendations to the MDCG. The group contributes to the development of proposals for guidance and common specifications in the field as referred to in Article 9 of MDR/Article 9 of the IVDR. The group elaborates proposals for the review of Commission Regulation (EU) 207/2012 on electronic instructions of use of medical devices. The group continuously performs screening of the available sources for identification of novel, emerging technologies which inherit medical/clinical potential. 2. Membership Members/observers to the group are experts appointed by Member States and third countries participating in the MDCG. Member States / third countries may appoint alternates. Appointments are not time-limited. Any changes in the appointment shall be notified to the Commission without delay. Stakeholders may participate in the open sessions of the group either in the capacity of observers or following ad hoc invitations, in accordance with the Rules of Procedure of the MDCG. 3. Operation The group operates in accordance with the terms and rules applicable to the MDCG, unless specified otherwise in these Terms of Reference. The group shall be chaired by a representative of the Commission. Where appropriate, it may be co-chaired by a member of the working group. The group shall report to the MDCG. The meetings are convened by the Chair. The group shall meet either in physical meetings or for audio- or videoconferences. Physical meetings of the group take place at least twice a year. Minutes on the discussion on each point on the agenda and on the positions delivered by the group shall be meaningful and complete. The group coordinates its activities with other MDCG working groups as   appropriate.
8. Eudamed – see the register of Expert Groups under the code E01309

9. Unique Device Identification (UDI) – Terms of reference

. Tasks and roles The group provides assistance to the MDCG on all issues related to introduction and operation of the Unique Device Identification system (UDI system) under Regulation (EU) 2017/745 on medical devices (MDR) and Regulation (EU) 2017/746 on in-vitro diagnostic medical devices (IVDR). The *group provides advice on all matters related to device identification and traceability, including implementation of the relevant provisions of the MDR on implant cards. In the field of its activities, the group prepares draft guidance for endorsement by the MDCG, or an input for the delegated acts foreseen in the MDR and IVDR. 2. Membership Members/observers to the group are experts appointed by Member States and third countries participating in the MDCG. Member States / third countries may appoint alternates. Appointments are not time-limited. Any changes in the appointment shall be notified to the Commission without delay. Stakeholders may participate in the open sessions of the group either in the capacity of observers or following ad hoc invitations, in accordance with the Rules of Procedure of the MDCG. 3. Operation The group operates in accordance with the terms and rules applicable to the MDCG, unless specified otherwise in these Terms of Reference. The group shall be chaired by a representative of the Commission. Where appropriate, it may be co-chaired by a member of the working group. The group shall report to the MDCG. The meetings are convened by the Chair. The group shall meet either in physical meetings or for audio- or videoconferences. Physical meetings of the group take place at least twice a year. Minutes on the discussion on each point on the agenda and on the positions delivered by the group shall be meaningful and complete. The group coordinates its activities with other MDCG working groups as appropriate.*

10. International Matters—Terms of reference

The Working Group on International Matters provides assistance to the MDCG on any international issues related to medical devices and in-vitro diagnostic medical devices, in particular, it monitors international regulation trends. In addition, the group coordinates the formulation of common views and positions of EU Member States on harmonisation topics discussed within the International Medical Device Regulators Forum (IMDRF). The activities of the group take into account the positions, recommendations, and any relevant documents prepared by other working groups of the MDCG.

11. In vitro diagnostic medical devices (IVD)—Terms of reference

The Working Group on In Vitro Diagnostic Medical Devices (IVD) provides assistance to the MDCG on all IVD specific issues, in particular, it develops and promotes homogenous application and implementation of Regulation (EU) 2017/746 (IVDR). It prepares draft guidance on IVD related issues for endorsement of the MDCG. The group coordinates its activities with other MDCG working groups as appropriate and, whenever needed, provides them with input on IVD specific aspects of their work (such as in the field of classification, performance studies, performance evaluation and post-market performance follow-up of IVDs).

European Regulations—MDR

MDR Classification system shall see several new rules added to the existing requirements. There is also the introduction of a new IVDR classification system (A, B, C, D) with 'A' representing the least risk and 'D' high risk. The new rules primarily relate to:

o   Software
o   Nanomaterials
o   Ingested products
o   Non-viable human tissues, cells and derivatives

The new regulations place additional responsibilities and obligations on all parties in the sector. The core purpose of the new regulation is the focus on increased availability of information on the identification, performance and safety of devices. A system called MDR–EUDAMED aims to facilitate a databank for medical devices.

Manufacturer
o   Article 10
o   Quality management system
o   Risk management
o   Clinical evaluation/PMCF
o   Continued updates
o   UDI and registration
o   Labelling and language
o   Incident reporting/FSCA
o   Obligation to act
o   Periodic reporting
o   Liability cover for damage compensation

Authorised Representatives (AR)

o   Article 11
o   AR within the EU
o   Written mandate— clear
o   tasks
o   AR legally accountable if the manufacturer fails to meet obligations

- o Responsible person

Person Responsible for Regulatory Compliance

- o Article 15
- o Demonstration of expertise
- o Available within the organisation
- o Applies to manufacturer and authorised representatives
- o Responsible for checking conformity of devices
- o Updates to technical documentation
- o PMS obligations

Regulation (EU) 2017/745 of The European Parliament and of the Council of 5th April 2017 on medical devices, amending Directive 2001/83/EC, Regulation (EC) No 178/2002 and Regulation (EC) No 1223/2009 and repealing Council Directives 90/385/EEC and 93/42/EEC.
(Reference- Official EU website)

https://eur-

lex.europa.eu/legalcontent/EN/TXT/PDF/?uri=CELEX:32017R0745&from=E

N

Structure Of MDR- 2017/745

The new MDR Rule (collection of Chapters and articles and annexees are summarised below for ease of reference. The full extent of chapters and articles are available freely via the EU MDR website **www.eumdr.com**

CHAPTER I -SCOPE AND DEFINITIONS

Article 1 Subject matter and scope
Article 2 Definitions
Article 3 Amendment of certain definitions
Article 4 Regulatory status of products

CHAPTER II—Making Available on the Market and Putting Into Service of Devices, Obligations

Article 5 Placing on the market and putting into service
Article 6 Distance sales
Article 7 Claims
Article 8 Use of harmonised standards
Article 9 Common specifications
Article 10 General obligations of manufacturers
Article 11 Authorised representative
Article 12 Change of authorised representative
Article 13 General obligations of importers
Article 14 General obligations of distributors
Article 15 Person responsible for regulatory compliance
Article 16 Cases in which obligations of manufacturers apply to importers, distributors or other persons
Article 17 Single-use devices and their reprocessing
Article 18 Implant card and information to be supplied to the patient with an implanted device
Article 19 EU declaration of conformity
Article 20 CE marking of conformity
Article 21 Devices for special purposes
Article 22 Systems and procedure packs
Article 23 Parts and components
Article 24 Free movement

CHAPTER III—Identification and Traceability of Devices, Registration of Devices and of Economic Operators, Summary of Safety and Clinical Performance, European Database on Medical Devices

Article 25 Identification within the supply chain
Article 26 Medical devices nomenclature
Article 27 Unique Device Identification system
Article 28 UDI database
Article 29 Registration of devices
Article 30 Electronic system for registration of economic operators

CHAPTER IV- NOTIFIED BODIES

CHAPTER V—Classification and Conformity Assessment

SECTION 1 Classification

SECTION 2-Conformity assessment

CHAPTER Vi—Clinical Evaluation and Clinical

Investigations

CHAPTER VII—Post-Market Surveillance, Vigilance and Market Surveillance Section 1 Post-Market Surveillance

SECTION 3—Market Surveillance

CHAPTER VIII—Cooperation Between Member States, Medical Device Coordination Group Expert Laboratories, Expert Panels and Device Registers

CHAPTER IX—Confidentiality, Data Protection, Funding and Penalties

CHAPTER X—Final Provisions

ANNEXEES

ANNEXE I GENERAL SAFETY AND PERFORMANCE REQUIREMENTS CHAPTER I GENERAL REQUIREMENTS

CHAPTER II REQUIREMENTS REGARDING DESIGN AND MANUFACTURE

CHAPTER III REQUIREMENTS REGARDING THE INFORMATION SUPPLIED WITH THE DEVICE

ANNEXE II TECHNICAL DOCUMENTATION

ANNEXE III TECHNICAL DOCUMENTATION ON POST-MARKET SURVEILLANCE

ANNEXE IV EU DECLARATION OF CONFORMITY

ANNEXE XV CLINICAL INVESTIGATIONS
ANNEXE XVI LIST OF GROUPS OF PRODUCTS WITHOUT
AN INTENDED MEDICAL PURPOSE REFERRED TO IN
ARTICLE 1(2)

Regulation (EU) 2017/746 Of The European Parliament and of
the Council of 5th April 2017 on in vitro diagnostic medical
devices, and repealing Council Directives 98/79/EC Commission
Decision 2010/227/EU.

https://eur-lex.europa.eu/legal-

content/EN/TXT/PDF/?uri=CELEX:32017R0746&from=EN

Medical device Regulation (MDR 2017/745) and Risk Management

MDR specifies that devices shall achieve *"performance intended by their manufacturer and shall be designed and manufactured in such a way that, during normal conditions of use, they are suitable for their intended purpose."*

They shall be safe and effective and shall not compromise the clinical condition or the safety of patients, or the safety and health of users or, where applicable, other persons,.

Any risks which may be associated with their use must result or constitute in *"acceptable risks when weighed against the benefits to the patient and are compatible with a high level of protection of health and safety, taking into account the generally acknowledged state of the art."*

Under the general safety and performance requirements (GSPR) device risk must be as low a possible and give due diligence to residual risks or in other words risks that remain after all possible risk reduction, control and mitigation. GSPR Annexe 1 Section 2 and 3 details the requirements on the risk-benefit ration and on risk management and the life cycle of risk management applied to products.

Definition of Risk (MDR 2017/745)

Risk defined means the combination of the probability of occurrence of harm and the severity of that harm.

GSPR Annexe I Section 3 of MDR 2017/745, Annexe I

The requirement in this Annexe to reduce risks as far as possible means the reduction of risks as far as possible without adversely affecting the benefit-risk ratio.

3. Manufacturers shall establish, implement, document and maintain a risk management system. Risk management shall be understood as a continuous iterative process throughout the entire life cycle of a device, requiring regular systematic updating. In carrying out risk management manufacturers shall:

> *(a) establish and document a risk management plan for each device;*
> *(b) identify and analyse the known and foreseeable hazards associated with each device;*
> *(c) estimate and evaluate the risks associated with, and occurring during, the intended use and during reasonably foreseeable misuse;*
> *(d) eliminate or control the risks referred to in point (c) in accordance with the requirements of Section 4;*

(e) evaluate the impact of information from the production phase and, in particular, from the post-market surveillance system, on hazards and the frequency of occurrence thereof, on estimates of their associated risks, as well as on the overall risk, benefit-risk ratio and risk acceptability; and
(f) based on the evaluation of the impact of the information referred to in point (e), if necessary amend control measures in line with the requirements of Section 4. 4. Risk control measures adopted by manufacturers for the design and manufacture of the devices shall conform to safety principles, taking account of the generally acknowledged state of the art.

To reduce risks, Manufacturers shall manage risks so that the residual risk associated with each hazard as well as the overall residual risk is judged acceptable. In selecting the most appropriate solutions, manufacturers shall, in the following order of priority:

(a) eliminate or reduce risks as far as possible through safe design and manufacture; where appropriate, take adequate protection measures, including alarms if necessary, in relation to risks that cannot be eliminated; and (c) provide information for safety (warnings/precautions/contra-indications) and, where appropriate, training to users.

Manufacturers shall inform users of any residual risks.

GSPR Annexe I MDR 2017/745, Section 5 States
In eliminating or reducing risks related to use error, the manufacturer shall:

(a) reduce as far as possible the risks related to the ergonomic features of the device and the environment in which the device is intended to be used (design for patient safety), and

(b) give consideration to the technical knowledge, experience, education, training and use environment, where applicable, and the medical and physical conditions of intended users (design for lay, professional, disabled or other users).

GSPR Annexe I MDR 2017/745 Section 6
The characteristics and performance of a device shall not be adversely affected to such a degree that the health or safety of the patient or the user and, where applicable, of other persons are compromised during the lifetime of the device, as indicated by the manufacturer when the device is subjected to the stresses which can occur during normal conditions of use and has been properly maintained per the manufacturer's instructions.

7. Devices shall be designed, manufactured and packaged in such a way that their characteristics and performance during their intended use are not adversely affected during transport and storage, for example, through fluctuations of temperature and humidity, taking account of the instructions and information provided by the manufacturer.
8. All known and foreseeable risks, and any undesirable side-effects, shall be minimised and be acceptable when weighed against the evaluated benefits to the patient and/or user arising from the achieved performance of the device during normal conditions of use.

9. For the devices referred to in Annexe XVI, the general safety requirements set out in Sections 1 and 8 shall be understood to mean that the device, when used under the conditions and for the purposes intended, does not present a risk at all or presents a risk that is no more than the maximum acceptable risk related to the product's use which is consistent with a high level of protection for the safety and health of persons.

Article 8 Use of Harmonised Standards 1

Devices that are in conformity with the relevant harmonised standards, or the relevant parts of those standards, the references of which have been published in the Official Journal of the European Union, shall be presumed to conform with the requirements of this regulation covered by those standards or parts thereof.

The first subparagraph shall also apply to system or process requirements to be fulfilled under this regulation by economic operators or sponsors, including those relating to quality management systems, risk management, post-market surveillance systems, clinical investigations, clinical evaluation or post-market clinical follow-up ('PMCF').

References in this regulation to harmonised standards shall be understood as meaning harmonised standards (references published in the Official Journal of the European Union).

References in this regulation to harmonised standards shall also include the monographs of the European Pharmacopoeia adopted by the Convention on the Elaboration of a European Pharmacopoeia, in particular on surgical sutures and on the interaction between medicinal products and materials used in devices containing such medicinal products, provided that references to those monographs have been published in the Official Journal of the European Union.

Article 8 Use of Harmonised Standards 1

Devices that are in conformity with the relevant harmonised standards, or the relevant parts of those standards, the references of which have been published in the Official Journal of the European Union, shall be presumed to conform with the requirements of this regulation covered by those standards or parts thereof.

The first subparagraph shall also apply to system or process requirements to be fulfilled in accordance with this regulation by economic operators or sponsors, including those relating to quality management systems, risk management, post-market surveillance systems, clinical investigations, clinical evaluation or post-market clinical follow-up ('PMCF').

References in this regulation to harmonised standards shall also include the monographs of the European Pharmacopoeia adopted under the Convention on the Elaboration of a European Pharmacopoeia, in particular on surgical sutures and on the interaction between medicinal products and materials used in devices containing such medicinal products, provided that references to those monographs have been published in the Official Journal of the European Union.

Manufacturer Responsibilities

Determine if your device is a medical device or a product without an intended medical purpose referred to in Annexe XVI.

Determine the classification of your device per the requirements of Chapter V and Annexe VIII, (Class I non-sterile, non-measuring and non-reusable surgical instrument medical devices and Class A in vitro medical devices do not require the intervention of a Notified Body).

Identify the general safety and performance requirements that apply to your device (s) per Annexe I.

Identify the harmonised standards and common specifications required to demonstrate compliance with the general safety and performance requirements applicable to your device(s).

Determine the conformity assessment route appropriate to your device(s) Annexes IX, X or XI as appropriate.

Determine the technical documentation required to demonstrate compliance with the general safety and performance requirements applicable to your device(s).

Develop your technical documentation in compliance with the above requirements per Annexe II.

Review your post-market surveillance, vigilance and market surveillance systems per the requirements of Chapter VII.

Develop your post-market technical documentation per the requirements of Annexe III.

Review your clinical evaluation and clinical investigations for compliance to Chapter VI 2017/745 for medical devices and clinical evidence, performance evaluation and performance studies for compliance to Chapter VI 2017/746 for in vitro diagnostic medical devices.

Review your clinical evaluation and post-market surveillance for compliance to Annexe XIV 2017/745 for medical devices and interventional clinical performance studies and certain other performance studies for compliance to Annexe XIV 2017/746 for in vitro diagnostic medical devices.

Review your clinical investigations per the requirements of Annexe XV 2017/745 for medical devices.

Draw up your declaration of conformity in compliance with Annexe IV.

Develop your UDI –DI and UDI-PI.

Obtain an SRN.

Apply to a duly designated notified body under regulation 2017/745 and/or 2017/746.

Notified Bodies

Re-evaluate the notified body quality management system in line with the requirements of 2017/745 and/or 2017/746.
Apply for designation under 2017/745 and/or 2017/746.
Liaise with the manufacturers to ensure a thorough understanding of the requirements by all economic operators.

MDR and Design Change/Design Management

Building upon the medical device directive and ISO 13485, MDR 2017/745 has detailed requirements in respect of design changes, their management and implementation. These requirements are detailed in the general safety and performance requirements (Annexe 1) Chapter 1 and also in Chapter 2—requirements regarding design and manufacture. The intended use of the device must be maintained when any design changes are required. Fundamentally, the safety and performance of the device must be demonstrated and maintained.

The section below (in italics) references the relevant content in MDR for Design under the General requirements in Annexe I, Chapter I and Chapter II

ANNEXE I

GENERAL SAFETY AND PERFORMANCE REQUIREMENTS

CHAPTER I *GENERAL REQUIREMENTS*

1. Devices shall achieve the performance intended by their manufacturer and shall be designed and manufactured in such a way that, during normal conditions of use, they are suitable for their intended purpose. They shall be safe and effective and shall not compromise the clinical condition or the safety of patients, or the safety and health of users or, where applicable, other persons, provided that any risks which may be associated with their use constitute acceptable risks when weighed against the benefits to the patient and are compatible with a high level of protection of health and safety, taking into account the generally acknowledged state of the art.

2. The requirement in this Annexe to reduce risks as far as possible means the reduction of risks as far as possible without adversely affecting the benefit-risk ratio.

3. Manufacturers shall establish, implement, document and maintain a risk management system.

Risk management shall be understood as a continuous iterative process throughout the entire life cycle of a device, requiring regular systematic updating. In carrying out risk management manufacturers shall:

(a) establish and document a risk management plan for each device;

(b) identify and analyse the known and foreseeable hazards associated with each device;

(c) estimate and evaluate the risks associated with, and occurring during, the intended use and during reasonably foreseeable misuse;

(d) eliminate or control the risks referred to in point (c) in accordance with the requirements of Section 4;

(e) evaluate the impact of information from the production phase and, in particular, from the post-market surveillance system, on hazards and the frequency of occurrence thereof, on estimates of their associated risks, as well as on the overall risk, benefit-risk ratio and risk acceptability; and

(f) based on the evaluation of the impact of the information referred to in point (e), if necessary amend control measures in line with the requirements of Section 4.

4. Risk control measures adopted by manufacturers for the design and manufacture of the devices shall conform to safety principles, taking account of the generally acknowledged state of the art. To reduce risks, Manufacturers shall manage risks so that the residual risk associated with each hazard as well as the overall residual risk is judged acceptable. In selecting the most appropriate solutions, manufacturers shall, in the following order of priority:

(a) eliminate or reduce risks as far as possible through safe design and manufacture;

(b) where appropriate, take adequate protection measures,

including alarms if necessary, in relation to risks that cannot be eliminated; and

(c) provide information for safety (warnings/precautions/contra-indications) and, where appropriate, training to users.

Manufacturers shall inform users of any residual risks.

5. In eliminating or reducing risks related to use error, the manufacturer shall:

(a) reduce as far as possible the risks related to the ergonomic features of the device and the environment in which the device is intended to be used (design for patient safety), and

(b) give consideration to the technical knowledge, experience, education, training and use environment, where applicable, and the medical and physical conditions of intended users (design for lay, professional, disabled or other users).

6. The characteristics and performance of a device shall not be adversely affected to such a degree that the health or safety of the patient or the user and, where applicable, of other persons are compromised during the lifetime of the device, as indicated by the manufacturer when the device is subjected to the stresses which can occur during normal conditions of use and has been properly maintained per the manufacturer's instructions.

7. Devices shall be designed, manufactured and packaged in such a way that their characteristics and performance during their intended use are not adversely affected during transport and storage, for example, through fluctuations of temperature and humidity, taking account of the instructions and information provided by the manufacturer.

8. All known and foreseeable risks, and any undesirable side-effects, shall be minimised and be acceptable when weighed against the evaluated benefits to the patient and/or user arising from the achieved performance of the device during normal conditions of use.

9. For the devices referred to in Annexe XVI, the general safety requirements set out in Sections 1 and 8 shall be understood to mean that the device, when used under the conditions and for the purposes intended, does not present a risk at all or presents a risk that is no more than the maximum acceptable risk related to the product's use which is consistent with a high level of protection for the safety and health of persons.

CHAPTER II

REQUIREMENTS REGARDING DESIGN AND MANUFACTURE

10. Chemical, physical and biological properties

10.1. Devices shall be designed and manufactured in such a way as to ensure that the characteristics and performance requirements referred to in Chapter I are fulfilled. Particular attention shall be paid to:

(a) the choice of materials and substances used, particularly as regards toxicity and, where relevant, flammability;

(b) the compatibility between the materials and substances used and biological tissues, cells and body fluids, taking account of the intended purpose of the device and, where relevant, absorption, distribution, metabolism and excretion;

(c) the compatibility between the different parts of a device which consists of more than one implantable part;

(d) the impact of processes on material properties;

(e) where appropriate, the results of biophysical or modelling research the validity of which has been demonstrated beforehand;

(f) the mechanical properties of the materials used, reflecting, where appropriate, matters such as strength, ductility, fracture resistance, wear resistance and fatigue resistance;

(g)   surface properties; and

(h) the confirmation that the device meets any defined chemical and/or physical specifications.

10.2. Devices shall be designed, manufactured and packaged in such a way as to minimise the risk posed by contaminants and residues to patients, taking account of the intended purpose of the device, and to the persons involved in the transport, storage and use of the devices. Particular attention shall be paid to tissues exposed to those contaminants and residues and to the duration and frequency of exposure.

10.3. Devices shall be designed and manufactured in such a way that they can be used safely with the materials and substances, including gases, with which they enter into contact during their intended use; if the devices are intended to administer medicinal products they shall be designed and manufactured in such a way as to be compatible with the medicinal products concerned in accordance with the provisions and restrictions governing those medicinal products and that the performance of both the medicinal products and of the devices is maintained in accordance with their respective indications and intended use.

10.4. Substances

10.4.1. Design and manufacture of Devices

Devices shall be designed and manufactured in such a way as to reduce as far as possible the risks posed by substances or particles, including wear debris, degradation products and processing residues, that may be released from the device.

Devices, or those parts thereof or those materials used therein that:

— are invasive and come into direct contact with the human body,

— (re)administer medicines, body-liquids or other substances, including gases, to/from the body, or

— transport or store such medicines, body fluids or substances,

including gases, to be (re)administered to the body,

shall only contain the following substances in a concentration that is above 0,1 % weight by weight (w/w) where justified pursuant to Section 10.4.2:

(a)*substances which are carcinogenic, mutagenic or toxic to reproduction ('CMR'), of category 1A or 1B, per Part 3 of Annexe VI to Regulation (EC) No 1272/2008 of the European Parliament and of the Council (¹), or*

(b)*substances having endocrine-disrupting properties for which there is scientific evidence of probable serious effects to human health and which are identified either in accordance with the procedure set out in Article 59 of Regulation (EC) No 1907/2006 of the European Parliament and of the Council (²) or, once a delegated act has been adopted by the Commission pursuant to the first subparagraph of Article 5(3) of Regulation (EU) No 528/2012 of the European Parliament and the Council (³), following the criteria that are relevant to human health amongst the criteria established therein.*

10.4.2. Justification regarding the presence of CMR and/or endocrine-disrupting substances

The justification for the presence of such substances shall be based upon:

(a) *an analysis and estimation of potential patient or user exposure to the substance;*

(b) *an analysis of possible alternative substances, materials or designs, including, where available, information about independent research, peer-reviewed studies, scientific opinions from relevant scientific committees and an analysis of the availability of such alternatives;*

(c) *argumentation as to why possible substance and/ or material substitutes, if available, or design changes, if feasible, are inappropriate in relation to maintaining the functionality, performance and the benefit-risk ratios of the product; including taking into account if the intended use of such devices includes treatment of children or treatment of pregnant or breastfeeding women or treatment of other patient groups considered particularly vulnerable to such substances and/or materials; and*

(d) *where applicable and available, the latest relevant scientific committee guidelines under Sections 10.4.3. and 10.4.4.*

10.4.3. Guidelines on Phthalates

For the purposes of Section 10.4., the Commission shall, as soon as possible and by 26 May 2018, provide the relevant scientific committee with a mandate to prepare guidelines that shall be ready before 26 May 2020. The mandate for the committee shall encompass at least a benefit-risk assessment of the presence of phthalates which belong to either of the groups of substances referred to in points (a) and (b) of Section 10.4.1. The benefit-risk assessment shall take into account the intended purpose and context of the use of the device, as well as any available alternative substances and alternative materials, designs or medical treatments. When deemed appropriate on the basis of the latest scientific evidence, but at least every five years, the guidelines shall be updated.

10.4.4. Guidelines on other CMR and Endocrine-Disrupting Substances

Subsequently, the Commission shall mandate the relevant scientific committee to prepare guidelines as referred to in Section 10.4.3. also for other substances referred to in points (a) and (b) of Section 10.4.1., where appropriate.

10.4.5. Labelling

Where devices, parts thereof or materials used therein as referred to in Section 10.4.1. contain substances referred to in points (a) or (b) of Section 10.4.1. in a concentration above 0,1 % weight by weight (w/w), the presence of those substances shall be labelled on the device itself and/or on the packaging for each unit or, where appropriate, on the sales packaging, with the list of such substances. If the intended use of such devices includes treatment of children or treatment of pregnant or breastfeeding women or treatment of other patient groups considered particularly vulnerable to such substances and/or materials, information on residual risks for those patient groups and, if applicable, on appropriate precautionary measures shall be given in the instructions for use.

10.5. Devices shall be designed and manufactured in such a way as to reduce as far as possible the risks posed by the unintentional ingress of substances into the device taking into account the device and the nature of the environment in which it is intended to be used.

10.6. Devices shall be designed and manufactured in such a way as to reduce as far as possible the risks linked to the size and the properties of particles which are or can be released into the patient's or user's body, unless they come into contact with intact skin only. Special attention shall be given to nanomaterials.

11. *Infection and Microbial Contamination*

11.1. Devices and their manufacturing processes shall be designed in such a way as to eliminate or to reduce as far as possible the risk of infection to patients, users and, where applicable, other persons. The design shall:

(a) reduce as far as possible and appropriate the risks from unintended cuts and pricks, such as needle stick injuries,

(b)   allow easy and safe handling,

(c) reduce as far as possible any microbial leakage from the device and/or microbial exposure during use, and

(d) prevent microbial contamination of the device or its content

such as specimens or fluids.

11.2. Where necessary devices shall be designed to facilitate their safe cleaning, disinfection, and/or re-sterilisation.

11.3. Devices labelled as having a specific microbial state shall be designed, manufactured and packaged to ensure that they remain in that state when placed on the market and remain so under the transport and storage conditions specified by the manufacturer.

11.4. Devices delivered in a sterile state shall be designed, manufactured and packaged in accordance with appropriate procedures, to ensure that they are sterile when placed on the market and that, unless the packaging which is intended to maintain their sterile condition is damaged, they remain sterile, under the transport and storage conditions specified by the manufacturer, until that packaging is opened at the point of use. It shall be ensured that the integrity of that packaging is clearly evident to the final user.

11.5. Devices labelled as sterile shall be processed, manufactured, packaged and, sterilised using appropriate, validated methods.

11.6. Devices intended to be sterilised shall be manufactured and packaged in appropriate and controlled conditions and facilities.

11.7. Packaging systems for non-sterile devices shall maintain the integrity and cleanliness of the product and, where the devices are to be sterilised before use, minimise the risk of microbial contamination; the packaging system shall be suitable taking account of the method of sterilisation indicated by the manufacturer.

11.8. The labelling of the device shall distinguish between identical or similar devices placed on the market in both a sterile and a non-sterile condition added to the symbol used to indicate that devices are sterile.

12. Devices incorporating a substance considered to be a medicinal product and devices that are composed of substances or of combinations of substances that are absorbed by or locally dispersed in the human body.

12.1. In the case of devices referred to in the first subparagraph of Article 1(8), the quality, safety and usefulness of the substance which, if used separately, would be considered to be a medicinal product within the meaning of point (2) of Article 1 of Directive 2001/83/EC, shall be verified by analogy with the methods specified in Annexe I to Directive 2001/83/EC, as required by the applicable conformity assessment procedure under this Regulation.

12.2. Devices that are composed of substances or of combinations of substances that are intended to be introduced into the human body, and that are absorbed by or locally dispersed in the human body shall comply, where applicable and in a manner limited to the aspects not covered by this Regulation, with the relevant requirements laid down in Annexe I to Directive 2001/83/EC for the evaluation of absorption, distribution, metabolism, excretion, local tolerance, toxicity, interaction with other devices, medicinal products or other substances and potential for adverse reactions, as required by the applicable conformity assessment procedure under this Regulation.

13. Devices Incorporating Materials of Biological Origin

13.1. For devices manufactured utilising derivatives of tissues or cells of human origin which are non-viable or are rendered non-viable covered by this Regulation in accordance with point (g) of Article 1(6), the following shall apply:

(a) donation, procurement and testing of the tissues and cells shall be done per Directive 2004/23/EC;

(b) processing, preservation and any other handling of those tissues and cells or their derivatives shall be carried out to provide safety for patients, users and, where applicable, other persons. In particular, safety with regard to viruses and other transmissible agents shall be addressed by

appropriate methods of sourcing and by implementation of validated methods of elimination or inactivation in the course of the manufacturing process;

(c) the traceability system for those devices shall be complementary and compatible with the traceability and data protection requirements laid down in Directive 2004/23/EC and in Directive 2002/98/EC.

13.2. For devices manufactured utilising tissues or cells of animal origin, or their derivatives, which are non-viable or rendered non-viable the following shall apply:

(a) where feasible taking into account the animal species, tissues and cells of animal origin, or their derivatives, shall originate from animals that have been subjected to veterinary controls that are adapted to the intended use of the tissues. Information on the geographical origin of the animals shall be retained by manufacturers;

(b) sourcing, processing, preservation, testing and handling of tissues, cells and substances of animal origin, or their derivatives, shall be carried out to provide safety for patients, users and, where applicable, other persons. In particular safety with regard to viruses and other transmissible agents shall be addressed by implementation of validated methods of elimination or viral inactivation in the course of the manufacturing process, except when the use of such methods would lead to unacceptable degradation compromising the clinical benefit of the device;

(c) in the case of devices manufactured utilising tissues or cells of animal origin, or their derivatives, as referred to in Regulation (EU) No 722/2012 the particular requirements laid down in that Regulation shall apply.

13.3. For devices manufactured utilising non-viable biological substances other than those referred to in Sections 13.1 and 13.2, the processing, preservation, testing and handling of those substances shall be carried out to provide safety for patients, users and, where applicable, other persons, including in the waste disposal chain. In particular, safety with regard to viruses and other transmissible agents shall be addressed by appropriate methods of sourcing and by implementation of validated methods of elimination or inactivation in the course of the manufacturing process.

14. Construction of Devices and Interaction with Their Environment

14.1. If the device is intended for use in combination with other devices or equipment the whole combination, including the connection system shall be safe and shall not impair the specified performance of the devices. Any restrictions on use applying to such combinations shall be indicated on the label and/or in the instructions for use. Connections which the user has to handle, such as fluid, gas transfer, electrical or mechanical coupling, shall be designed and constructed in such a way as to minimise all possible risks, such as misconnection.

14.2. Devices shall be designed and manufactured in such a way as to remove or reduce as far as possible:

(a) the risk of injury, in connection with their physical features, including the volume/pressure ratio, dimensional and where appropriate ergonomic features;

(b) risks connected with reasonably foreseeable external influences or environmental conditions, such as magnetic fields, external electrical and electromagnetic effects, electrostatic discharge, radiation associated with diagnostic or therapeutic procedures, pressure, humidity, temperature, variations in pressure and acceleration or radio signal interferences;

(c) the risks associated with the use of the device when it comes into contact with materials, liquids, and substances,

including gases, to which it is exposed during normal conditions of use;

(d) the risks associated with the possible negative interaction between software and the IT environment within which it operates and interacts;

(e) the risks of accidental ingress of substances into the device;

(f) the risks of reciprocal interference with other devices normally used in the investigations or for the treatment given; and

(g) risks arising where maintenance or calibration are not possible (as with implants), from ageing of materials used or loss of accuracy of any measuring or control mechanism.

14.3. Devices shall be designed and manufactured in such a way as to minimise the risks of fire or explosion during normal use and in single fault condition. Particular attention shall be paid to devices the intended use of which includes exposure to or use in association with flammable or explosive substances or substances which could cause combustion.

14.4. Devices shall be designed and manufactured in such a way that adjustment, calibration, and maintenance can be done safely and effectively.

14.5. Devices that are intended to be operated together with other devices or products shall be designed and manufactured in such a way that the interoperability and compatibility are reliable and safe.

14.6 Any measurement, monitoring or display scale shall be designed and manufactured in line with ergonomic principles, taking account of the intended purpose, users and the environmental conditions in which the devices are intended to be used.

14.7.   Devices shall be designed and manufactured in such a way as to facilitate their safe disposal and the safe disposal of related waste substances by the user, patient or other person. To that end, manufacturers shall identify and test procedures and measures as a result of which their devices can be safely disposed after use. Such procedures shall be described in the instructions for use.

15.   Devices with a Diagnostic or Measuring Function

15.1.   Diagnostic devices and devices with a measuring function, shall be designed and manufactured in such a way as to provide sufficient accuracy, precision and stability for their intended purpose, based on appropriate scientific and technical methods. The limits of accuracy shall be indicated by the manufacturer.

15.2.   The measurements made by devices with a measuring function shall be expressed in legal units conforming to the provisions of Council Directive 80/181/EEC (⁴).

16.   Protection against Radiation

16.1.   General

(a) Devices shall be designed, manufactured and packaged in such a way that exposure of patients, users and other persons to radiation is reduced as far as possible, and in a manner that is compatible with the intended purpose, whilst not restricting the application of appropriate specified levels for therapeutic and diagnostic purposes.

(b) The operating instructions for devices emitting hazardous or potentially hazardous radiation shall contain detailed information as to the nature of the emitted radiation, the means of protecting the patient and the user, and on ways of avoiding misuse and of reducing the risks inherent to installation as far as possible and appropriate. Information regarding the acceptance and performance testing, the acceptance criteria, and the maintenance procedure shall also be specified.

16.2. Intended Radiation

(a) Where devices are designed to emit hazardous, or potentially hazardous, levels of ionising and/or non-ionising radiation necessary for a specific medical purpose the benefit of which is considered to outweigh the risks inherent to the emission, it shall be possible for the user to control the emissions. Such devices shall be designed and manufactured to ensure reproducibility of relevant variable parameters within an acceptable tolerance.

(b) Where devices are intended to emit hazardous, or potentially hazardous, ionising and/or non-ionising radiation, they shall be fitted, where possible, with visual displays and/or audible warnings of such emissions.

16.3. Devices shall be designed and manufactured in such a way that exposure of patients, users and other persons to the emission of unintended, stray or scattered radiation is reduced as far as possible. Where possible and appropriate, methods shall be selected which reduce the exposure to radiation of patients, users and other persons who may be affected.

16.4. Ionising Radiation

(a) Devices intended to emit ionising radiation shall be designed and manufactured taking into account the requirements of the Directive 2013/59/Euratom laying down basic safety standards for protection against the dangers arising from exposure to ionising radiation.

(b) Devices intended to emit ionising radiation shall be designed and manufactured in such a way as to ensure that, where possible, taking into account the intended use, the quantity, geometry and quality of the radiation emitted can be varied and controlled, and, if possible, monitored during treatment.

(c) Devices emitting ionising radiation intended for diagnostic radiology shall be designed and manufactured in such a way as to achieve an image and/or output quality that are *appropriate to the intended medical purpose whilst minimising radiation exposure of the patient and user.*

(d) Devices that emit ionising radiation and are intended for therapeutic radiology shall be designed and manufactured in such a way as to enable reliable monitoring and control of the delivered dose, the beam type, energy and, where appropriate, the quality of radiation.

17. Electronic programmable systems—devices that incorporate electronic programmable systems and software that are devices in themselves

17.1. Devices that incorporate electronic programmable systems, including software, or software that are devices in themselves, shall be designed to ensure repeatability, reliability and performance in line with their intended use. In the event of a single fault condition, appropriate means shall be adopted to eliminate or reduce as far as possible consequent risks or impairment of performance.

17.2. For devices that incorporate software or for software that are devices in themselves, the software shall be developed and manufactured in accordance with the state of the art taking into account the principles of development, life cycle, risk management, including information security, verification and validation.

17.3. Software referred to in this Section that is intended to be used in combination with mobile computing platforms shall be designed and manufactured taking into account the specific features of the mobile platform (e.g. size and contrast ratio of the screen) and the external factors related to their use (varying environment as regards the level of light or noise).

17.4. Manufacturers shall set out minimum requirements concerning hardware, IT networks characteristics and IT security measures, including protection against unauthorised access, necessary to run the software as intended.

18. Active Devices and Devices Connected to Them

18.1. For non-implantable active devices, in the event of a single fault condition, appropriate means shall be adopted to eliminate or reduce as far as possible consequent risks.

18.2. Devices where the safety of the patient depends on an internal power supply shall be equipped with a means of determining the state of the power supply and an appropriate warning or indication for when the capacity of the power supply becomes critical. If necessary, such warning or indication shall be given prior to the power supply becoming critical.

18.3. Devices where the safety of the patient depends on an external power supply shall include an alarm system to signal any power failure.

18.4. Devices intended to monitor one or more clinical parameters of a patient shall be equipped with appropriate alarm systems to alert the user of situations which could lead to death or severe deterioration of the patient's state of health.

18.5. Devices shall be designed and manufactured in such a way as to reduce as far as possible the risks of creating electromagnetic interference which could impair the operation of the device in question or other devices or equipment in the intended environment.

18.6. Devices shall be designed and manufactured in such a way as to provide a level of intrinsic immunity to electromagnetic interference such that is adequate to enable them to operate as intended.

18.7. Devices shall be designed and manufactured in such a way as to avoid, as far as possible, the risk of accidental electric shocks to the patient, user or any other person, both during normal use of the device and in the event of a single fault condition in the device, provided the device is installed and maintained as indicated by the manufacturer.

18.8. Devices shall be designed and manufactured in such a way as to protect, as far as possible, against unauthorised access that could hamper the device from functioning as intended.

19. Particular Requirements for Active Implantable Devices

19.1. Active implantable devices shall be designed and manufactured in such a way as to remove or minimise as far as possible:

(a) risks connected with the use of energy sources with particular reference, where electricity is used, to insulation, leakage currents and overheating of the devices,

(b) risks connected with medical treatment, in particular those resulting from the use of defibrillators or high-frequency surgical equipment, and

(c) risks which may arise where maintenance and calibration are impossible, including:

— *excessive increase of leakage currents,*

— *ageing of the materials used,*

— *excess heat generated by the device,*

—*decreased accuracy of any measuring or control mechanism.*

19.2. Active implantable devices shall be designed and manufactured in such a way as to ensure

—*if applicable, the compatibility of the devices with the substances they are intended to administer, and*

— *the reliability of the source of energy.*

19.3. Active implantable devices and, if appropriate, their component parts shall be identifiable to allow any necessary measure to be taken following the discovery of a potential risk in connection with the devices or their component parts.

19.4. Active implantable devices shall bear a code by which they and their manufacturer can be unequivocally identified (particularly with regard to the type of device and its year of manufacture); it shall be possible to read this code, if necessary, without the need for a surgical operation.

20. Protection Against Mechanical and Thermal Risks

20.1. Devices shall be designed and manufactured in such a way as to protect patients and users against mechanical risks connected with, for example, resistance to movement, instability and moving parts.

20.2. Devices shall be designed and manufactured in such a way as to reduce to the lowest possible level the risks arising from vibration generated by the devices, taking account of technical progress and of the means available for limiting vibrations, particularly at source, unless the vibrations are part of the specified performance.

20.3. Devices shall be designed and manufactured in such a way as to reduce to the lowest possible level the risks arising from the noise emitted, taking account of technical progress and of the means available to reduce noise, particularly at source, unless the noise emitted is part of the specified performance.

20.4. Terminals and connectors to the electricity, gas or hydraulic and pneumatic energy supplies which the user or other person has to handle, shall be designed and constructed in such a way as to minimise all possible risks.

20.5. Errors likely to be made when fitting or refitting certain parts which could be a source of risk shall be made impossible by the design and construction of such parts or, failing this, by information given on the parts themselves and/or their housings.

The same information shall be given on moving parts and/or their housings where the direction of movement needs to be known to avoid risk.

20.6. Accessible parts of devices (excluding the parts or areas intended to supply heat or reach given temperatures) and their surroundings shall not attain potentially dangerous temperatures under normal conditions of use.

21. Protection Against the Risks Posed to the Patient or User by Devices Supplying Energy or Substances

21.1. Devices for supplying the patient with energy or substances shall be designed and constructed in such a way that the amount to be delivered can be set and maintained accurately enough to ensure the safety of the patient and of the user.

21.2. Devices shall be fitted with the means of preventing and/or indicating any inadequacies in the amount of energy delivered or substances delivered which could pose a danger. Devices shall incorporate suitable means to prevent, as far as possible, the accidental release of dangerous levels of energy or substances from an energy and/or substance source.

21.3. The function of the controls and indicators shall be clearly specified on the devices. Where a device bears instructions required for its operation or indicates operating or adjustment parameters by means of a visual system, such information shall be understandable to the user and, as appropriate, the patient.

22. Protection Against the Risks Posed by Medical Devices Intended by the Manufacturer for Use by Lay Persons

22.1. Devices for use by lay persons shall be designed and manufactured in such a way that they perform appropriately for their intended purpose taking into account the skills and the means available to lay persons and the influence resulting from variation that can be reasonably anticipated in the lay person's technique and environment. The information and instructions provided by the manufacturer shall be easy for the lay person to understand and apply.

22.2. Devices for use by lay persons shall be designed and manufactured in such a way as to:

—ensure that the device can be used safely and accurately by the intended user at all stages of the procedure, if necessary after appropriate training and/or information,

—reduce, as far as possible and appropriate, the risk from unintended cuts and pricks such as needle stick injuries, and

—reduce as far as possible the risk of error by the intended user in the handling of the device and, if applicable, in the interpretation of the results.

22.3. Devices for use by lay persons shall, where appropriate, include a procedure by which the lay person:

—can verify that, at the time of use, the device will perform as intended by the manufacturer, and

—if applicable, is warned if the device has failed to provide a valid result.

CHAPTER III

REQUIREMENTS REGARDING THE INFORMATION SUPPLIED WITH THE DEVICE

23. Label and Instructions for Use

23.1. General Requirements Regarding the Information Supplied by the Manufacturer

Each device shall be accompanied by the information needed to identify the device and its manufacturer, and by any safety and performance information relevant to the user, or any other person, as appropriate. Such information may appear on the device itself, on the packaging or in the instructions for use, and shall, if the manufacturer has a website, be made available and kept up to date on the website, taking into account the following:

(a) The medium, format, content, legibility, and location of the label and instructions for use shall be appropriate to the particular device, its intended purpose and the technical knowledge, experience, education or training of the intended user(s). In particular, instructions for use shall be written in terms readily understood by the intended user and, where appropriate, supplemented with drawings and diagrams.

(b) *The information required on the label shall be provided on the device itself. If this is not practicable or appropriate, some or all of the information may appear on the packaging for each unit, and/or on the packaging of multiple devices.*

(c) *Labels shall be provided in a human-readable format and may be supplemented by machine-readable information, such as radio-frequency identification ('RFID') or bar codes.*

(d) *Instructions for use shall be provided together with devices. By way of exception, instructions for use shall not be required for class I and class IIa devices if such devices can be used safely without any such instructions and unless otherwise provided for elsewhere in this Section.*

(e) *Where multiple devices are supplied to a single user and/or location, a single copy of the instructions for use may be provided if so agreed by the purchaser who in any case may request further copies to be provided free of charge.*

(f) *Instructions for use may be provided to the user in non-paper format (e.g. electronic) to the extent, and only under the conditions, set out in Regulation (EU) No 207/2012 or in any subsequent implementing rules adopted pursuant to this Regulation.*

(g) *Residual risks which are required to be communicated to the user and/or other person shall be included as limitations, contraindications, precautions or warnings in the information supplied by the manufacturer.*

(h) *Where appropriate, the information supplied by the manufacturer shall take the form of internationally recognised symbols. Any symbol or identification colour used shall conform to the harmonised standards or CS. In areas for which no harmonised standards or CS exist, the symbols and colours shall be described in the documentation supplied with the device.*

23.2. Information on the Label

The label shall bear all of the following particulars:

(a) the name or trade name of the device;

(b) the details strictly necessary for a user to identify the device, the contents of the packaging and, where it is not obvious for the user, the intended purpose of the device;

(c) the name, registered trade name or registered trademark of the manufacturer and the address of its registered place of business;

(d) if the manufacturer has its registered place of business outside the Union, the name of the authorised representative and address of the registered place of business of the authorised representative;

(e) where applicable, an indication that the device contains or incorporates:

—a medicinal substance, including human blood or plasma derivative, or

—tissues or cells, or their derivatives, of human origin, or

—tissues or cells of animal origin, or their derivatives, as referred to in Regulation (EU) No 722/2012;

(f) where applicable, information labelled in accordance with Section 10.4.5.;

(g) the lot number or the serial number of the device preceded by the words LOT NUMBER or SERIAL NUMBER or an equivalent symbol, as appropriate;

(h) the UDI carrier referred to in Article 27(4) and Part C of Annexe VII;

(i) an unambiguous indication of t the time limit for using or implanting the device safely, expressed at least in terms of year and month, where this is relevant;

(j) where there is no indication of the date until when it may be used safely, the date of manufacture. This date of manufacture may be included as part of the lot number or serial number, provided the date is clearly identifiable;

(k) an indication of any special storage and/or handling condition that applies;

(l) if the device is supplied sterile, an indication of its sterile state and the sterilisation method;

(m) warnings or precautions to be taken that need to be brought to the immediate attention of the user of the device, and to any other person. This information may be kept to a minimum in which case more detailed information shall appear in the instructions for use, taking into account the intended users;

(n) if the device is intended for single-use, an indication of that fact. A manufacturer's indication of single-use shall be consistent across the Union;

(o) if the device is a single-use device that has been reprocessed, an indication of that fact, the number of reprocessing cycles already performed, and any limitation as regards the number of reprocessing cycles;

(p) if the device is custom-made, the words 'custom-made device';

(q) an indication that the device is a medical device. If the device is intended for clinical investigation only, the words 'exclusively for clinical investigation';

(r) in the case of devices that are composed of substances or of combinations of substances that are intended to be introduced into the human body via a body orifice or applied to the skin and that are absorbed by or locally dispersed in the human body, the overall qualitative composition of the device and quantitative information on the main constituent or constituents responsible for achieving the principal *intended action;*

(s) for active implantable devices, the serial number, and for other implantable devices, the serial number or the lot number.

23.3. Information on the Packaging Which Maintains the Sterile Condition of a Device ('Sterile Packaging')

The following particulars shall appear on the sterile packaging:

(a) an indication permitting the sterile packaging to be recognised as such,

(b) a declaration that the device is in a sterile condition,

(c)   the method of sterilisation,

(d) the name and address of the manufacturer,

(e)   a description of the device,

(f) if the device is intended for clinical investigations, the words 'exclusively for clinical investigations',

(g) if the device is custom-made, the words 'custom-made device',

(h)   the month and year of manufacture,

(i) an unambiguous indication of the time limit for using or implanting the device safely expressed at least in terms of year and month, and

(j) an instruction to check the instructions for use for what to do if the sterile packaging is damaged or unintentionally opened before use.

23.4. Information in the Instructions for Use

The instructions for use shall contain all of the following particulars:

(a) the particulars referred to in points (a), (c), (e), (f), (k), (l),

(n) and (r) of Section 23.2;

(b) the device's intended purpose with a clear specification of indications, contra-indications, the patient target group or groups, and of the intended users, as appropriate;

(c) where applicable, a specification of the clinical benefits to be expected.

(d) where applicable, links to the summary of safety and clinical performance referred to in Article 32;

(e) the performance characteristics of the device;

(f) where applicable, information allowing the healthcare professional to verify if the device is suitable and select the corresponding software and accessories;

(g) any residual risks, contraindications and any undesirable side-effects, including information to be conveyed to the patient in this regard;

(h) specifications the user requires to use the device appropriately, e.g. if the device has a measuring function, the degree of accuracy claimed for it;

(i) details of any preparatory treatment or handling of the device before it is ready for use or during its use, such as sterilisation, final assembly, calibration, etc., including the levels of disinfection required to ensure patient safety and all available methods for achieving those levels of disinfection;

(j) any requirements for special facilities, or special training, or particular qualifications of the device user and/or other persons;

(k) the information needed to verify whether the device is properly installed and is ready to perform safely and as intended by the manufacturer, together with, where relevant:

—details of the nature, and frequency, of preventive and regular maintenance, and of any preparatory cleaning or

disinfection,

—identification of any consumable components and how to replace them,

—information on any necessary calibration to ensure that the device operates properly and safely during its intended lifetime, and

—methods for eliminating the risks encountered by persons involved in installing, calibrating or servicing devices;

(l) if the device is supplied sterile, instructions in the event of the sterile packaging being damaged or unintentionally opened before use;

(m) if the device is supplied non-sterile with the intention that it is sterilised before use, the appropriate instructions for sterilisation;

(n) if the device is reusable, information on the appropriate processes for allowing reuse, including cleaning, disinfection, packaging and, where appropriate, the validated method of re-sterilisation appropriate to the Member State or Member States in which the device has been placed on the market. Information shall be provided to identify when the device should no longer be reused, e.g. signs of material degradation or the maximum number of allowable reuses;

(o) an indication, if appropriate, that a device can be reused only if it is reconditioned under the responsibility of the manufacturer to comply with the general safety and performance requirements;

(p) if the device bears an indication that it is for single-use, information on known characteristics and technical factors known to the manufacturer that could pose a risk if the device were to be re-used. This information shall be based on a specific section of the manufacturer's risk management documentation, where such characteristics and technical factors shall be addressed in detail. If in accordance with point (d) of Section 23.1. no instructions for use are required, this information shall be made available to the user upon request;

(q) for devices intended for use together with other devices and/or general-purpose equipment:

—information to identify such devices or equipment, to obtain a safe combination, and/or

—information on any known restrictions to combinations of devices and equipment;

(r) if the device emits radiation for medical purposes:

—detailed information as to the nature, type and where appropriate, the intensity and distribution of the emitted radiation,

—the means of protecting the patient, user, or other person from unintended radiation during use of the device;

(s) information that allows the user and/or patient to be informed of any warnings, precautions, contra-indications, measures to be taken and limitations of use regarding the device. That information shall, where relevant, allow the user to brief the patient about any warnings, precautions, contra-indications, measures to be taken and limitations of use regarding the device. The information shall cover, where appropriate:

—warnings, precautions and/or measures to be taken in the event of malfunction of the device or changes in its performance that may affect safety,

—warnings, precautions and/or measures to be taken as regards the exposure to reasonably foreseeable external influences or environmental conditions, such as magnetic fields, external electrical and electromagnetic effects, electrostatic discharge, radiation associated with diagnostic or therapeutic procedures, pressure, humidity, or temperature,

—warnings, precautions and/or measures to be taken as

regards the risks of interference posed by the reasonably foreseeable presence of the device during specific diagnostic investigations, evaluations, or therapeutic treatment or other procedures such as electromagnetic interference emitted by the device affecting other equipment,

—if the device is intended to administer medicinal products, tissues or cells of human or animal origin, or their derivatives, or biological substances, any limitations or incompatibility in the choice of substances to be delivered,

—warnings, precautions and/or limitations related to the medicinal substance or biological material that is incorporated into the device as an integral part of the device; and

—precautions related to materials incorporated into the device that contain or consist of CMR substances or endocrine-disrupting substances, or that could result in sensitisation or an allergic reaction by the patient or user;

(t) in the case of devices that are composed of substances or of combinations of substances that are intended to be introduced into the human body and that are absorbed by or locally dispersed in the human body, warnings and precautions, where appropriate, related to the general profile of interaction of the device and its products of metabolism with other devices, medicinal products and other substances as well as contra-indications, undesirable side-effects and risks relating to overdose;

(u) in the case of implantable devices, the overall qualitative and quantitative information on the materials and substances to which patients can be exposed;

(v) warnings or precautions to be taken to facilitate the safe disposal of the device, its accessories and the consumables used with it, if any. This information shall cover, where appropriate:

—infection or microbial hazards such as explants, needles or surgical equipment contaminated with potentially infectious substances of human origin, and

— physical hazards such as from sharps.

If in accordance with the point (d) of Section 23.1 no instructions for use are required, this information shall be made available to the user upon request;

(w) for devices intended for use by lay persons, the circumstances in which the user should consult a healthcare professional;

(x) for the devices covered by this Regulation pursuant to Article 1(2), information regarding the absence of a clinical benefit and the risks related to use of the device;

(y) date of issue of the instructions for use or, if they have been revised, date of issue and identifier of the latest revision of the instructions for use;

(z) a notice to the user and/or patient that any serious incident that has occurred in relation to the device should be reported to the manufacturer and the competent authority of the Member State in which the user and/or patient is established;

(aa) information to be supplied to the patient with an implanted device in accordance with Article 18;

(ab) for devices that incorporate electronic programmable systems, including software, or software that are devices in themselves, minimum requirements concerning hardware, IT networks characteristics and IT security measures, including protection against unauthorised access, necessary to run the software as intended.

(^{1}) *Regulation (EC) No 1272/2008 of the European Parliament and of the Council of 16 December 2008 on classification, labelling and packaging of substances and mixtures, amending and repealing Directives 67/548/EEC and 1999/45/EC, and amending Regulation (EC) No 1907/2006* **(OJ L 353, 31.12.2008, p. 1)**.

(^{2}) *Regulation (EC) No 1907/2006 of the European Parliament and of the Council of 18 December 2006 concerning the Registration, Evaluation, Authorisation and Restriction of Chemicals (REACH)* **(OJ L 396, 30.12.2006, p. 1)**.

(^{3}) *Regulation (EU) No 528/2012 of the European Parliament and the Council of 22 May 2012 concerning the making available on the market of and use of biocidal products* **(OJ L 167, 27.6.2012, p. 1)**.

(^{4}) *Council Directive 80/181/EEC of 20 December 1979 on the approximation of the laws of the Member States relating to units of measurement and on the repeal of Directive 71/354/EEC* **(OJ L 39, 15.2.1980, p. 40)**.

CE marking

Article 17, and affix the CE marking of conformity in accordance with Article 18

Article 17
EU declaration of conformity
1. *The EU declaration of conformity shall state that the requirements specified in this Regulation have been fulfilled. The manufacturer shall continuously update the EU declaration of conformity. The EU declaration of conformity shall, as a minimum, contain the information set out in Annexe IV and shall be translated into an official Union language or languages required by the Member State(s) in which the device is made available.*

2. Where, concerning aspects not covered by this Regulation, devices are subject to other Union legislation which also requires an EU declaration of conformity by the manufacturer that fulfilment of the requirements of that legislation has been demonstrated, a single EU declaration of conformity shall be drawn up in respect of all Union acts applicable to the device. The declaration shall contain all the information required for identification of the Union legislation to which the declaration relates.

3. By drawing up the EU declaration of conformity, the manufacturer shall assume responsibility for compliance with the requirements of this Regulation and all other Union legislation applicable to the device.

4. The Commission is empowered to adopt delegated acts in accordance with Article 108 amending the minimum content of the EU declaration of conformity set out in Annexe IV in the light of technical progress.

Article 18

CE marking of conformity

1. Devices, other than devices for performance studies, considered to be in conformity with the requirements of this Regulation shall bear the CE marking of conformity, as presented in Annexe V.

2. The CE marking shall be subject to the general principles set out in Article 30 of Regulation (EC) No 765/2008.

3. The CE marking shall be affixed visibly, legibly and indelibly to the device or its sterile packaging. Where such affixing is not possible or not warranted on account of the nature of the device, the CE marking shall be affixed to the packaging. The CE marking shall also appear in any instructions for use and on any sales packaging.

4. The CE marking shall be affixed before the device is placed on the market. It may be followed by a pictogram or any other mark indicating a special risk or use.

5. *Where applicable, the CE marking shall be followed by the identification number of the notified body responsible for the conformity assessment procedures set out in Article 48. The identification number shall also be indicated in any promotional material which mentions that a device fulfils the requirements for CE marking.*
6. *Where devices are subject to other Union legislation which also provides for the affixing of the CE marking, the CE marking shall indicate that the devices also fulfil the requirements of that other legislation.*

Ref: **https://eur-lex.europa.eu/legal-content/EN/TXT/?uri=CELEX%3A32017R0746**

ANNEXE IV

EU DECLARATION OF CONFORMITY

The EU declaration of conformity shall contain the following information:

1. Name, registered trade name or registered trademark and, if already issued, SRN referred to in Article 28 of the manufacturer, and, if applicable, its authorised representative, and the address of their registered place of business where they can be contacted and their location be established;

2. A statement that the EU declaration of conformity is issued under the sole responsibility of the manufacturer;

3. The Basic UDI-DI as referred to in Part C of Annexe VI;

4. Product and trade name, product code, catalogue number or other unambiguous reference allowing identification and traceability of the device covered by the EU declaration of conformity, such as a photograph, where appropriate, as well as its intended purpose. Except for the product or trade name, the information allowing identification and traceability may be provided by the Basic UDI-DI referred to in point 3;

5. Risk class of the device in accordance with the rules set out in Annexe VIII;

6. A statement that the device that is covered by the present declaration conforms with this Regulation and, if applicable, with any other relevant Union legislation that provides for the issuing of an EU declaration of conformity;

7. References to any CS used and in relation to which conformity is declared;

8. Where applicable, the name and identification number of the notified body, a description of the conformity assessment procedure performed and identification of the certificate or certificates issued;

9. Where applicable, additional information;

10. Place and date of issue of the declaration, name and function of the person who signed it as well as an indication for, and on behalf of whom, that person signed, signature.

ANNEXE V—CE MARKING OF CONFORMITY

1. The CE marking shall consist of the initials 'CE' taking the following form:

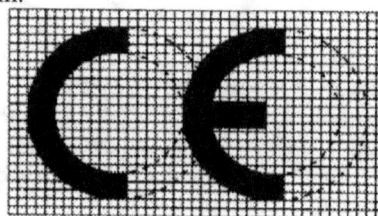

2. If the CE marking is reduced or enlarged the proportions given in the above graduated drawing shall be respected.

3. The various components of the CE marking shall have substantially the same vertical dimension, which may not be less than 5 mm. This minimum dimension may be waived for small-scale devices.

UDI system referred to in Article 24 and with the registration obligations referred to in Article 26 and 28.

APPENDIX 1

Regulation (EU) 2017/745 -Listed summary of Chapters and articles

Regulation (EU) 2017/745 of The European Parliament and of the Council of 5th April 2017 on medical devices, amending Directive 2001/83/EC, Regulation (EC) No 178/2002 and Regulation (EC) No 1223/2009 and repealing Council Directives 90/385/EEC and 93/42/EEC.

CHAPTER I—SCOPE AND DEFINITIONS

CHAPTER II—MAKING AVAILABLE ON THE MARKET AND PUTTING INTO SERVICE OF DEVICES, OBLIG

CHAPTER III—IDENTIFICATION AND TRACEABILITY OF DEVICES, REGISTRATION OF DEVICES AND OF ECONOMIC OPERATORS, SUMMARY OF SAFETY AND CLINICAL PERFORMANCE, EUROPEAN DATABASE ON MEDICAL DEVICES

CHAPTER IV—NOTIFIED BODIES

CHAPTER V—CLASSIFICATION AND CONFORMITY

ASSESSMENT SECTION 1 Classification

CHAPTER II IMPLEMENTING RULES
CHAPTER III CLASSIFICATION RULES

ANNEXE IX CONFORMITY ASSESSMENT BASED ON A
QUALITY MANAGEMENT SYSTEM AND ON ASSESSMENT OF
TECHNICAL DOCUMENTATION

ANNEXE X CONFORMITY ASSESSMENT BASED ON TYPE-
EXAMINATION

ANNEXE XI CONFORMITY ASSESSMENT BASED ON PRODUCT
CONFORMITY VERIFICATION

ANNEXE XII CERTIFICATES ISSUED BY A NOTIFIED BODY

ANNEXE XIII PROCEDURE FOR CUSTOM-MADE DEVICES

ANNEXE XIV CLINICAL EVALUATION AND POST-MARKET
CLINICAL FOLLOW-UP

ANNEXE XV CLINICAL INVESTIGATIONS
ANNEXE XVI LIST OF GROUPS OF PRODUCTS WITHOUT AN
INTENDED MEDICAL PURPOSE REFERRED TO IN ARTICLE 1(2)

www.ingramcontent.com/pod-product-compliance
Lightning Source LLC
Chambersburg PA
CBHW070600220526
45467CB00003B/1254